TABLE OF CONTENTS

To my parents, Hannah and Colin, who brought me into this world, gave me a wonderful upbringing, and who still provide amazing support so I can devote the time to complete a project like this.

To my husband, Tim, who gives constructive criticism when it's needed, unconditional love in abundance, and who is the best father I can ever imagine.

To my two sons, Ben and Toby, who will always be the most divine things I have ever achieved.

To all the women who pick up this book and strive to keep healthy and fit, YOU are truly inspirational.

Acknowledgements

My heartfelt thanks to each of the following people who have generously provided valuable input into this book. I am truly grateful for their contributions and support.

* Michele Robinson (photographer extraordinaire)
* Dr Dereck Souter (obstetrician extraordinaire)
* Dr Richard Fisher (fertility specialist extraordinaire)

Also:

* Fertility Associates for permission to reproduce information on the IVF process and related photographs
* physiotherapists
  Michelle Booth (reviewed the postnatal material)
  Maree Frost (reviewed the pelvic floor material)
  Karen Donaldson (reviewed the crucial core and pilates material)

* programme participants
  Mandy McPhail
  Michele Grimmond
  Mandy Hampton

* researchers interviewed
Dr Jennifer Ann Kruger
Sarah Hopkins

* others: Dr Bill Hummel, Nicola Wood, Toni Marsh, Louise Pagonis.

Foreword

Dereck Souter
FRCOG
FRANZCOG
DDU
Obstetrician
Gynaecologist

It is with great pleasure that I am writing a foreword to what is likely to become the defining book of exercise in pregnancy. Suzy has created not only an exercise manual for pregnancy, but also an excellent guide on coping with the various stresses and strains on both the body and mind that are part of a normal pregnancy.

It is increasingly being said that pregnancy is a test of the body for life, with conditions such as high blood pressure and diabetes occurring for the first time in pregnancy, once thought to be confined to pregnancy, being quite likely to recur in later life. With this in mind, pregnancy is an ideal time for a woman to start reviewing her lifestyle and diet to ensure that not only a good pass in the test of pregnancy is achieved, but also that the basis of a healthy lifestyle is established.

This book provides a realistic, balanced exercise programme for pregnancy, acknowledging that pregnancy can have a significant effect on energy levels and that there will be both good days and bad days. Guidance for coping with the bad days is also given.

In my experience as a specialist obstetrician I have seen how different the experience of pregnancy can be between women, and even how for individual women each pregnancy can be so different. Not everything in pregnancy is able to be controlled by the mother, and even in the womb babies often seem to have a mind and a timetable of their own. However, although mothers and their caregivers cannot control or guarantee the outcomes of pregnancy, we can both influence them. You may not have a pregnancy that allows you to achieve every exercise, or even exercise as often as recommended in this book, but it will provide a useful guide on keeping as healthy during the pregnancy and how to return as close as you can to your pre-pregnancy body as quickly as possible.

Suzy is to be congratulated on writing an excellent book on looking after yourself in pregnancy and also providing some frank personal insights on her experiences of pregnancy and childbirth. I wish you the reader the healthiest of pregnancies.

Dereck Souter

Foreword

Dr Richard Fisher
CNZM
FRANZCOG
CREI
Specialist in Reproductive
Medicine

It is my pleasure to provide a foreword for this book. Suzy shares both her professional wisdom and her personal insights into pregnancy in a way which integrates the professional and the personal extraordinarily well. Her personal journey has been complicated, but a calm sense of reality, coupled with an ever-present optimism, has enabled her to reflect on this journey in a way which is helpful for others.

As a day-to-day guide for staying fit and healthy throughout pregnancy, with its clearly proven benefits to the outcome for your child, this book will be a handy companion. As a source of inspiration to couples distressed by their difficulty in conceiving, it will be a talisman. Not everyone who follows Suzy's advice or history will be as lucky in the end as she and Tim have been. All, however, will know they have done everything they reasonably can to work with the vagaries of nature.
Richard Fisher

Introduction

Mature mums

There is no doubt that women in the Western world are on average having children later in life. Choosing to become a parent in your thirties or forties is part of an established upward trend. Across OECD countries the average age at which women have their first child has increased from 24 years in the 1970s to 28 years in 2009.

More specifically it is 27.8 years for New Zealanders, 28 years for Australians and first-time mums in the United Kingdom top the chart with an average age of 30.

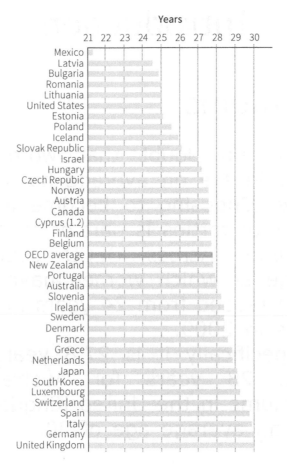

Fig.0.1: Source: OECD, Family Database

So, since the 1970s first-time maternal age has been increasing. Why?

Women are choosing briefcases over bassinets as they strive to accomplish personal goals and career objectives, complete tertiary study or seek increased financial stability. IVF techniques also contribute to women of an older age giving birth. It could also be simply down to finding the right partner—they're not always apparent when your eggs are at their prime.

Physically the optimum time for a woman to have a baby is in her twenties, when she has plenty of energy as well as the life skills to cope with being a mum. However, there is a lot to be said for becoming a mum in the decades that follow: more emotional maturity, more settled and more worldly (after having probably travelled or at very least experienced more of life), more financially stable and more willing to make the necessary sacrifices that having a baby inevitability involves. Crayon on the walls or paint on the carpet are definitely annoying, but can be treated with a perspective that comes from relaxing about the 'immaculate' house you probably once ran.

Take me, for example. I am 45 and a mother of two, but I didn't have my first child until I was 39—definitely delayed compared with the median age of New Zealand women giving birth. There are of course risks that come with being pregnant over the age of 35; for example, increased risk of miscarriage, gestational diabetes, conditions involving high blood pressure, chromosomal abnormalities, and the sheer weight of biological statistics are against you in terms of fertility.

And what about your physical body? As you get older, isn't it harder to bounce back from being pregnant? Sure, you have to work at it rather than rely on youthful resilience, but, armed with the information and skills contained in this book, I firmly believe you will be able to keep age where it belongs—in the mind, and in perspective. As Abraham Lincoln once said: 'In the end, it's not the years in your life that count, it's the life in your years.' You are as old as you feel, and striving for a healthy, active pregnancy will keep you young in spirit.

You are pregnant—congratulations!

This is one of the most exciting journeys you will ever take in your life. If you are on to your second, third or more baby, you are now nodding your head with a wealth of understanding and appreciation for how amazing the human body truly is. How adaptable, how resilient and how magnificent it really is in every sense. If this is your first pregnancy, then it is a unique and incredibly exciting time, full of discovery and wonder at how your body is slowly but surely growing another human being inside.

Every pregnant woman's journey is different and specific to her. The information in this book is a general guide, summarising the latest research and giving sensible safe options and information about exercising throughout pregnancy as part of a healthy lifestyle for you and your baby. It is designed to provide you with the tools to enjoy and revel in your changing body over the nine months' gestation and three months following the birth. It is not a guide to losing significant weight or gaining a high level of fitness. There is a time and a place for everything, and pregnancy is not the time to have those goals in mind.

Let me keep it real right from the get-go. I am not all rose-tinted glasses when it comes to pregnancy. Nausea, back ache and feeling the size of a whale are just some of those lovely pregnancy accompaniments that each woman, to varying extents, has to accommodate and learn to tolerate. Mother Nature is a potent force, though, and her ability to make you forget the uncomfortable bits and focus on the positives should not be underestimated. This no doubt accounts for why we so willingly do it all again, some many times over.

One part of the journey in writing this book I did not foresee was the difficulty I encountered in having a second child. My first pregnancy had been fairly textbook: easy conception, normal pregnancy, fast birth and a fairly typical recovery. This probably lulled me into a false sense of fertility security around falling pregnant a second time. True to form I did initially conceive easily, but I miscarried and what then followed was a three-year tumultuous journey through multiple IVF cycles and another miscarriage before we finally had our second child—our little miracle baby. I have written about my experiences of miscarriage and IVF through this time, and you will find that chapter towards the end of the book.

Mums who have had their first child after 35 share their experiences

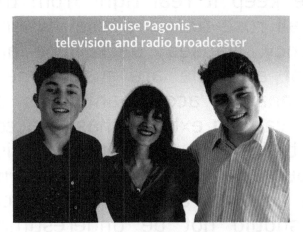

I was lucky enough to have my first baby Oliver at 38 without any real problems, but had to wait until I was 43 before my second long-awaited son, William, arrived. Those intervening five years were extremely stressful. I endured five miscarriages, and a threatened early labour at 25 weeks, after which I was told to take it easy—I wasn't even allowed to go swimming. I still remember it was one of the most humid summers on record and I had to watch people in swim suits walk past the house on their way to the local beach while I sweltered at home trying to rest. However, it did pay off, as William was born at 37 weeks. Both boys have brought me much joy and happiness.

I had always been fit and active, enjoying biking, swimming, and regular walks. Aside from the short period of enforced rest, I maintained most activities while I was pregnant. During my first pregnancy I also discovered aqua-natal classes which were great for meeting other pregnant mums. I think doing regular exercise helped me get back in shape fairly quickly after birth. A good walk was a great way of getting rid of that feeling of being shut off from the world—especially if I added in a nice coffee break! I never felt I was an 'older mum', as my first antenatal group was full of women like me. I met my husband when I was 36 so there was no chance of having a baby any earlier.

Overall, being older with young kids has been great! I had the chance to achieve a lot in my broadcasting career before having children, which paved the way for now doing lots of different part-time roles, and I love still having a teenager at home. I would encourage mums having babies later in life after being career-driven to join as many groups as possible, because there is so much networking you can still do with little ones in tow, and many opportunities can come from that. These days I have joined a gym and go at least three times a week, as well as cycling and taking my kayak out on the harbour. I love doing different kinds of exercise, and I think the best thing when you are pregnant is to find an activity you like and do it as often as you can—even better, go with a friend and motivate each other.

Toni Marsh – former television weather presenter

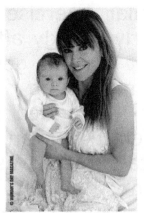

Having been through a cancer scare and told I probably couldn't have kids, being informed by my doctor that I was pregnant at 40 was a huge surprise. Nothing, however, was put on the back-burner because of it. Being a regular gym-goer from way back, I worked out through my entire pregnancy, and was back at the gym after the requisite six weeks following a C-section.

Of course I took things a little easier and listened to my body as well as advice from my obstetrician, but, as I discovered, age is definitely no barrier to producing a happy,

> healthy baby so long as you are happy and healthy yourself.

So why should you be health aware and consider exercise during this nine-month journey? Most mothers want to give their baby the very best start in life. We all yearn for healthy, happy babies, and, unless you have medical complications, making moderate exercise a regular part of your pregnancy gives both you and your baby a head start in the health stakes.

Closely following the desire to do the best by your growing baby is a new mum's concern about her ballooning in size over nine months. While there is nothing more beautiful and vital than a healthy pregnant woman showing all the physical signs and exhibiting a full round belly that is evidence of that growing baby inside, many woman struggle with all the extra weight gain and shape change that goes with it. Exercise can be your friend: preventing excessive weight gain—particularly from mid-pregnancy on—and helping you regain your pre-pregnancy shape more quickly.

The normal range of weight gain for pregnancy is 10–15 kilograms. Research shows that those women who have been exercising prior to pregnancy and continue doing so throughout their pregnancies can affect their amount of weight gain, determining how much of that weight is fat, and whether they are likely to hang on to that pregnancy-accumulated fat. In some studies the weight difference between those who exercised and those who did not equated to around three kilograms. Not that much, you might say, but when it is three kilograms of fat, well, that can make a fairly significant difference in how a pregnant woman looks and, equally important, how she feels about herself. Women who have not exercised prior to pregnancy but who start a regular regime during or after their first trimester can also influence their weight gain and fatty deposits. However, studies revealed a significant effect only if the amount of exercise added up to about three hours total a week. For example, that might be 30 minutes on six days a week, or 45 minutes on four days a week.

While it is hard to quantify, most women report that exercising regularly throughout pregnancy helps them maintain a positive attitude and feel good about themselves, and alleviates the worry of 'will I ever get back to what I was like before?' Maybe it is because getting out and being active proves to the mum-to-be that pregnancy is a natural state and not one of which to be fearful. A sense of achievement also goes a long way to boosting self-esteem and helping a pregnant woman feel positive about the upcoming huge change to her lifestyle.

Introducing or maintaining exercise throughout the three trimesters can be the catalyst to making better healthy choices, but exercise is not the only factor when it comes to achieving a healthy pregnancy: what you eat and how much you rest and relax also have a huge influence. The overall aim is to keep fit. So for some of you that will mean introducing exercise in the first place; for others, it's a case of keeping on with what you have been doing but with modifications in each trimester. For those who are already very active, it is likely to mean adjusting to a far less intense routine. Pregnancy is a natural condition, not an illness, so unless you have a high-risk pregnancy it should be possible and enjoyable to exercise throughout most of it.

As an older mum (35 years or older), you may be wondering whether your age will affect your pregnancy and birth. It's possible that you will have extra tests and more attentive care from your lead maternity carer (LMC) simply because of your age, but in most cases this is purely precautionary. Older women can and do have perfectly healthy pregnancies. Being in an older age bracket can also mean your body is not as fit and nubile as it once was! Maybe you get more aches and twinges? Maybe your energy levels aren't as high? Regardless of your current age and condition, the advice and programmes presented in this book will help you navigate a sensible and resilient pathway through the three trimesters and the first three months after birth.

The best way to use this book

❋ If you are yet to be pregnant or are currently in the **first trimester,** read all of the material up to and including the **first trimester,** and then follow the subsequent chapters as your pregnancy progresses.

❋ If you are in the **second trimester,** read chapters 1–4, then skip to the **second trimester** for specifics on what you should do, and follow the subsequent chapters.

❋ If you are in the **third trimester,** read chapters 1–4, then skip to the **third trimester** for specifics on what you should do, and follow the subsequent chapters.

❋ If you read this book from cover to cover, you will encounter some repetition with regard to safety considerations and exercise prescription. This is deliberate, to ensure that all readers are well informed and kept safe.

Let's get started!

Chapter 1

Getting Started

Safety first

Regardless of your current fitness level, you should discuss your intention to participate in regular physical activity with your doctor, midwife or obstetrician. This is not scaremongering—just sound practical advice. Your lead maternity caregiver (LMC) is an infinite source of wisdom when it comes to growing healthy babies, and should be your first port of call if you have any doubts or concerns as regards your general pregnancy and staying active. In order to do their job well, they need to have the complete picture of how your pregnancy is progressing. Being fit, eating healthily and taking time out when you feel tired is part of that overall picture. You, together with your health-care team will make the best decisions about your care when everything is fully disclosed. Your LMC can advise you if there are any particular modifications you may need to make, but most likely they'll be championing your positive attitude to maintaining the good health and wellbeing of both you and your baby over the nine months and beyond.

> *In Australia and New Zealand we refer to our main maternity caregiver, be that an obstetrician or midwife (as is usually the case), as the LMC—lead maternity carer. The term 'LMC' will be used throughout the book, and relates to the person who is monitoring and tracking your pregnancy throughout the nine months, and who most likely will be there when you go into labour and deliver.*

A great idea is to get into the habit of keeping an exercise diary, for you and your LMC to review. It saves you having to remember what you did and when, and acts as a good self-motivator. An example of a simple chart, which you can use as the basis on which construct your own, is given opposite (Fig.1.1).

Blowing traditional advice out the window

In years gone by, doctors advised women to 'rest up' when they discovered they were expecting. The main concerns were that exercising would raise body temperature which might cause congenital abnormalities, and that the need for oxygenated blood by the exercising muscles would *steal* the supply away from the developing baby. It sounds like pretty scary stuff. However, this historical advice was based on studies in the 1970s and 1980s which subjected laboratory animals to hard physical exertion combined with under-nutrition, and has subsequently been shown to have been far too conservative.

Day	Mode	Duration	Intensity	How I Felt
Monday	Power walk	40 mins	Brisk: hills and flat	Comfortable. Should add more hills for challenge.
Tuesday				
Wednesday				
Thursday				
Friday				
Saturday				
Sunday				

Fig 1.1

What the research says

A review of the national exercise guidelines for pregnant women throughout New Zealand, Australia, the United Kingdom, the USA and Canada overwhelmingly concludes it is beneficial to exercise before, during and after pregnancy. 'Before' allows you to enter your pregnancy in the best possible state; 'during' helps you prepare physically and psychologically for the demands of labour, childbirth and the rigours of looking after a new baby, and achieve appropriate weight gain; and 'after' aids your postpartum recovery and gets you back into shape.

My first labour lasted a grand total of four and a half hours from the first twinge to the almighty pop! But, before you curse me as being lucky, let me tell you that this was both good and bad. Good in that it was over relatively quickly; bad in that it was fast and furious and gave my body very little time to stretch and get ready to eject a pumpkin through a key hole! However, the moral of the story is that I had exercised regularly throughout my first pregnancy, so in my case perhaps my being fit contributed to my shorter labour time. No promises, though!

These 'authorities' have progressed even further in recent years, with official recommendations going from merely saying that, yes, it is fine for pregnant women to exercise, to actively encouraging all women without contraindications to participate in aerobic and strength conditioning exercises as part of a healthy lifestyle during pregnancy.

Many common pregnancy complaints like—I'm tired/my veins are swollen—I now have *cankles* not ankles/I can't sleep at night/I'm stressed and worried—are reduced or alleviated in women who exercise. Furthermore, something that is bound to attract your keen attention: there is even some evidence that weight-bearing exercise—something as simple as regular, fast walking throughout your pregnancy—can reduce the length of labour and decrease delivery complications.

For the mother

Recent studies of regular exercise during pregnancy reveal:

❋ **NO** increase in: early pregnancy loss, late pregnancy complications, abnormal fetal growth or adverse neonatal outcomes

❋ **NO** link or association between pregnant women exercising and miscarriage, congenital malformations, ectopic pregnancies, pre-term rupture of membranes, placental insufficiency, retarded intrauterine growth, or unexplained fetal deaths

❋ **fewer** medical interventions during labour and delivery, and in some cases shorter labour times

❋ **decreased** rates of postpartum depression

❋ **enhancement** of the baby's birth weight

❋ **maintenance** and improvement of the mother's heart and blood vessels

❋ **improved** strength for regular lifting and carrying required with a newborn

 * **stronger** back muscles to counteract the pull and strain on your back and ligaments, as your centre of gravity shifts

 * **better** posture which prevents or alleviates some of the niggling complaints associated with pregnancy, particularly back pain

 * **better** awareness of the pelvic floor muscle exercises, helping prevent incontinence postpartum

 * **improved** positive mental attitude, helping the mother accept her changing body shape, and promoting self-esteem and confidence

 * **increased** resistance to fatigue

 * **better** quality sleep and better ability to deal with insomnia

 * **smaller** gain of extra body fat—outside of normal weight gain during pregnancy of 10–15 kilograms

 * **faster** recuperation after labour, and a more rapid return to pre-pregnancy fitness, body shape and a healthy weight

 * **reduced** chances of gestational diabetes which affects 5% of pregnant women resulting from the effects of hormones but which usually subsides after delivery (if you do have gestational diabetes, exercise helps improve your blood sugar levels)

 * **reduced** varicose veins and swelling of the feet and ankles

∗ **improved** calcium uptake by the body which helps prevent future osteoporosis.

The research goes further, too, emphasising the risks of NOT participating in exercise during pregnancy. In other words, here's what you risk by *not* being active:

∗ **loss** of muscular and cardiovascular fitness

∗ **excessive** maternal weight gain

∗ **higher** risk of gestational diabetes or pregnancy-induced hypertension

∗ **development** of varicose veins and deep vein thrombosis

∗ **higher** incidence of back pain

∗ **tougher** time adjusting mentally to the physical changes of pregnancy.

For the baby

Does exercising potentially affect the growing baby at different stages of pregnancy or during labour and birth? The consensus of the studies conducted is that babies of exercising mums are more resilient in the womb and more 'tough' when it came to the normal stresses associated with being born. When scientists looked at whether the *type* of exercise, the *duration* and the *intensity* affected the baby's vital signs during pregnancy, they found that the responses matched the exercise level: low level = low response, higher level = higher response. Importantly, the higher-level responses were within safe and normal limits unless the exercise was extreme.

During labour, babies born to exercising mums again were more resilient to the usual stresses and did not exhibit as many warning signs requiring attention or intervention during the birth process.

While the newborns of exercising mums tend to be a little leaner at birth, this does not affect their ability to thrive. In fact, they are often ahead on the charts when it comes to adapting easily to things in their new environment and settling themselves when disturbed.

It is not written up as research as yet, but there are suggestions from researchers that the newborns of women who exercise have perhaps been exposed to more stimuli and mild stresses—for example, sound and vibration—and that this has encouraged enhanced fetal development. In other words, adaptations learnt in the womb translate into a more resilient baby who is better able to deal with life outside in the big, bright world.

Any long-term benefits?

Long-term studies on the physical and mental development in infants and children born to exercising mums have yet to be concluded, but they are underway to track whether there are any sustained, positive and lasting effects. To date there are certainly no downsides or negative outcomes for the fetus, baby or growing child from having a mum who has continued exercising throughout her pregnancy.

In a nutshell

In uncomplicated pregnancies, women who are already active or who want to get active should be encouraged to participate in regular modified aerobic and strength conditioning exercises as part of a healthy lifestyle for mother and baby.

> An 'uncomplicated pregnancy' is one where neither the woman nor the developing baby have any significant health issues.

Miscarriage and exercise

The reality is that the words 'miscarriage' and 'exercise' should not appear in a sentence that implies any association. There is no link or research to show that regular moderate exercise during early pregnancy has any effect on the incidence of either miscarriage or birth defects. Spontaneous miscarriage occurs so frequently that, unless a woman has three in a row, it is not considered abnormal.

There has been much rumour, conjecture and misinformation that the physical effects of exercise early on in pregnancy will cause such things as ectopic pregnancy, miscarriage, or defects in the developing baby. There is no science to support this. It is wrong. Healthy women can continue on with their usual exercise when they plan to conceive or during early pregnancy, and those choosing to begin an exercise programme can do so without concern, provided that it is gradually introduced and is moderate in intensity.

Of course if you are bleeding and are threatening to miscarry, you should rest and consult your LMC, as physical activity is not advisable if you have a partially detached placenta.

Level of exercise

Staying active or becoming active and exercising moderately on most if not all days of the week will bring about a swathe of positive health benefits during your pregnancy. How would you like to have increased energy, improved mood and posture, better sleep, enhanced muscle-tone strength and endurance? Are you ready to sign on the dotted line? Of course you are—who wouldn't be?

For previously inactive pregnant women, three sessions per week of 15 minutes' duration is an excellent start. Then, over the course of a month, they can build up to the level for previously active women: 30–60 minutes on most if not all days of the week. Later in the book I will explain how to modify this standard prescription for each trimester, and give you plenty of safe exercise options.

Beginner—15 minutes, three times a week

Previously active—30–60 minutes most days of the week

I aim for a healthy lifestyle most of the time. The way I do this when I am not pregnant is by adhering to my achievable 90/10 Rule. It's something I came up with over a decade ago that keeps me motivated to consistently make healthy choices, but also realistically allows for life's ebb and flow. Here is how it goes: 90% of the time you keep yourself on track with your fitness goals and healthy eating; 10% of the time you cut yourself some slack and allow for the inevitable parties, dinners out, and days when family outings need to take priority over exercising.

However, just as exercise goals need to be adapted for pregnancy, so too does my 90/10 rule. For pregnant women an achievable motivational target is to aim for 80/20. Healthy pregnancy: 80% of the time keep yourself on track with activity, healthy food choices and a balance of relaxation, 20% of the time you cut yourself some slack and allow for those busy days, bouts of tiredness and blob-outs.

> *80/20 Rule: 80% of the time keep yourself on track, 20% of the time cut yourself some slack. Have a big-picture attitude to achieving a healthy pregnancy.*

A level-headed approach

The aim of exercise during pregnancy is to stay fit, or, if you have previously been sedentary, to gain some moderate fitness. It is *not* to achieve peak fitness, train for athletic competition or lose weight. Like you, most pregnant women are deeply committed to providing their unborn child with the best possible environment in which to grow. Once educated about any risks, a pregnant woman will go out of her way to minimise harm to the growing fetus. Moderate regular exercise, good nutrition, avoiding smoking, alcohol and drugs are behaviours that will indisputably give your new baby the chance it deserves.

Contraindications and risks

Get clearance first

There appears to be different schools of thought on what constitutes an absolute contraindication to exercising while pregnant *(don't do it)* and what is a condition that should be discussed with your LMC. In the interests of safety, these tables err on the conservative side, so if you have any of the conditions that are listed below and you are keen on maintaining or introducing some form of exercise, then please discuss it fully with your LMC. In consultation with you they will be able to point out the risks versus the benefits for your particular circumstances, and if appropriate will suggest suitable modifications or at very least put you in contact with someone qualified who can advise you on what you *are* able to achieve.

Contraindications to exercise

Absolute contraindications

If you have any of these conditions, your LMC will be on alert and so should you:

* serious heart disease or respiratory disease
* pre-eclampsia/pregnancy-induced high blood pressure
* premature labour during current pregnancy
* incompetent cervix
* multiple fetuses
* placenta previa after 28 weeks

* persistent second- or third-trimester bleeding
 * ruptured membranes
 * restrictive lung disease
 * growth-restricted fetus
 * uncontrolled type 1 diabetes.

Potential contraindications

Conditions where it is recommended your exercise regime be monitored by your LMC or health-care professional, as the risk to you or your baby might outweigh the benefits of exercise, include:
 * anaemia
 * previous spontaneous abortion
 * previous pre-term birth
 * mild heart or lung disease
 * multiple pregnancy in the third trimester.

If you do have any of the above, then discuss with your LMC what sort of exercise might be possible. Perhaps regular gentle walking or a stretch programme might be something achievable for you. It is worth asking, as in many cases just doing something is better than doing nothing.

Warning signs during exercise

If you experience any of these symptoms during exercise, stop the activity and discuss it with your LMC:

* excessive shortness of breath
* headache or dizziness
* pain—chest or abdominal pain in particular
* nausea or vomiting
* vaginal bleeding
* contractions
* deep back or pubic pain
* cramping in the lower abdomen
* sudden swelling of hands, face and ankles
* unusual change in the baby's movements—particularly a marked decrease in movement
* amniotic fluid leakage.

High-risk activities to avoid

These are activities where the risks outweigh any potential benefit from being active, whether throughout your pregnancy or at specific times in it.

Throughout your entire pregnancy, avoid:

✗ scuba diving—as your baby has no protection against decompression sickness and gas embolism under water.

In the first trimester the fetus is growing in a space within the mother's pelvis and so is essentially protected from injury. But as the pregnancy continues the fetus moves up and out as it grows, making it more susceptible to an injury from impact. Moreover, increasingly from the second trimester on, your expanding baby bump and altered centre of gravity both combine to make you more prone to falls. So say 'no thanks' to:

× parachuting
× waterskiing
× martial arts
× gymnastics
× horse riding
× downhill skiing.

All of these activities have an increased chance of potential injury to you and your baby; it's just not worth the risk.

Change, change, change

Pregnancy—'a natural growth state'—brings about changes and positive adaptations with your heart, lungs, hormones, blood flow, muscles ligaments and bones. Let us look at the main body changes that happen during pregnancy and how they relate to exercise, and then answer some common questions.

Changes to circulation and blood flow

The entire circulatory system changes dramatically during pregnancy to support the needs of both the growing fetus and the mother. Not only does exercising not work against any of these normal pregnancy adaptations, it actually aids them. The normal blood-flow changes that occur with regular weight-bearing exercise complement the blood-flow changes in pregnancy.

Early pregnancy symptoms—light-headedness, nausea, fatigue, cravings, constipation, bloating, and increased urine leading to frequent peeing—while annoying to put up with, often indicate changes that signal a healthy pregnancy.

Hormones released early on in pregnancy make blood vessels able to stretch more, so they need more fluid to fill them. For a while, until the body adapts to this new needed volume of blood, there will be a shortfall or 'underfill'. Consequently, a pregnant woman may experience some or all of the symptoms that accompany this state: waves of fatigue, racing pulse, nausea, pallor, sweating, and dizziness when getting up suddenly. Thankfully, by about the second trimester the body has adapted to this new state, with blood volume and cardiac output increasing by about 40%, and so the symptoms diminish or disappear.

The body also channels more blood flow to the skin, kidneys and reproductive organs. This is a good change that benefits the mother and fetus, but the side-effects felt are flushed palms and face. This may account for that often talked about 'pregnancy glow'.

Pregnant women are physiologically better able to dissipate body heat. They sweat more easily, which allows heat loss; have increased blood flow to the skin, allowing further heat loss; and the body's resting temperature decreases slightly.

These are all excellent physical adaptations to counteract the state of exercising while pregnant which are both heat generators. You may have read or heard of concerns about not getting hot when you are pregnant. This is likely to be based on research which showed 'a prolonged rise in core body temperature above 39.2° Celsius could disturb the growth and development of your baby'. Note the words 'prolonged' and 'could'. There used to be a lot of well-meaning but not scientifically based worry about pregnant women getting hot. The accepted practice now is to avoid getting too hot for any length of time and to keep well hydrated, especially in the first trimester.

There is virtually no chance of you overheating if you participate in *moderate* exercise. The only caution is if exercise is performed *intensely,* for a *prolonged* time, or in a *hot and humid* environment that you are not used to. So avoid the sweaty hot sessions of Bikram yoga, and give the sauna a miss. If you are suddenly in a tropical island climate, you should drop your exercise intensity considerably. Soaking in spa pools can also raise your body temperature, so in general it is advisable to avoid them. Dress for exercise in layers so you can peel off a level of clothing as you heat up.

Changes to breathing

While pregnant, your body's natural response is to breathe more deeply and take in more air so that the delivery of oxygen to the tissues of both mother and baby is improved. That said, pregnant women often feel breathless. Why is this? This is a normal response to a normal increase in a hormone called 'progesterone' which causes 'over-breathing'. Again, it is perfectly normal and just one of those quirky side-effects of being pregnant. Towards the end of pregnancy, the baby's size may make you feel as though your capacity to breathe is reduced, but studies indicate there is nothing to worry about as your lungs are functioning at normal or even improved levels.

The placenta, which acts as the baby's lung, is positively affected by exercise. The placentas of women who regularly exercise during early and mid-pregnancy grow faster and function better compared with those of women who don't, particularly in the second trimester.

Levels of oxygenated blood to baby during exercise

Many mothers worry that their baby will not receive enough oxygenated blood while they exercise. However, if you stick to the recommended guidelines for each trimester and don't overdo it, baby will be fine. The research recommends not exercising for longer than 90 minutes at more than 80% of your maximum heart rate; more than that *could* affect the amount of oxygenated blood available to the baby.

When *exercising,* the body naturally targets the blood flow towards the heart, muscles and skin. When *pregnant,* the body naturally increases blood flow to the reproductive organs, kidneys and skin. It may sound like a potential conflict, but there is enough oxygenated blood supply when a pregnant mum is exercising at a *moderate* level to adequately cater for both the exercising muscles and the baby.

If you stick to moderate exercise, then the only situation in which there is a risk of depleting the supply of oxygenated blood to the baby is at high altitudes—when there is decreased blood flow to the womb. At altitudes of over 2500 metres you should avoid exercising until you have acclimatised, which may take a few days.

Changes to muscles ligaments and bones

Regular exercise can ease or eliminate some of the most common pregnancy complaints like lower back pain and leg cramps. Maintaining strength in the back muscles, good posture and abdominal muscle tone helps to counteract body twinges, aches and niggles due to inevitable protrusion of your belly moving up and out as the pregnancy progresses.

Working out your fitness level

To work out the sort of programme you can follow throughout each trimester, it is important to get clear on your *current* level of fitness.

1. Have you done little or no exercise for months?

   Walking round the supermarket is about as good as it gets.

2. Do you participate in regular recreational exercise?

   I manage on average three to five sessions a week.

3. Are you regularly exercising to a high intensity?

   I do high-impact aerobics classes, or an activity like squash, five to seven days a week.

4. Are you a competitive athlete or do you play contact sports regularly?

   Do you classify yourself as being in group 1 or group 3? Then welcome to group 2, as this should be your exercise goal for the next nine months, with modifications as your pregnancy progresses. Even if you are a beginner, and your pregnancy is proceeding without complications, you can aim for three to five sessions a week. Remember, you will make those sessions achievable and specific to you by moderating how long and how hard you exercise.

Intensity of exercise

Whether it is aerobic-type exercise, strength training or stretching that you are performing while pregnant, the same word applies regarding the intensity of your endeavours to keep you safe and your workout effective: *moderate.*

With strength-training exercises, being able to complete a set of 8–15 repetitions should mean that the resistance is at a moderate level. With stretching you should apply all the usual self-checks to make sure you are in the correct position and alignment, but don't push the stretch position too hard, just take the muscle to the point of being stretched moderately and maintain that. Due to the ligament-softening hormone 'relaxin' that is present during pregnancy, avoid forcing your body into a stretch position as overstretching can cause lax ligaments and injury.

With aerobic or cardiovascular training you will need to be aware of the exertion of your heart and lungs. Aerobic activity is any steady, uninterrupted exercise that uses the large muscles of the body for a sustained period of time; for example, jogging, fast walking, cycling, swimming and some group fitness gym classes. The word 'aerobic' means 'with oxygen'. When you do this sort of exercise your heart rate and breathing rate increase, but in order to get the fitness benefits you need to get up a sweat for a decent length of time. The duration of your workout is easy enough to figure by counting increments of 5 minutes, a beginner attempting perhaps 15 minutes and an established exerciser probably aiming for 30–60 minutes.

Intensity is usually measured by taking your heart rate as an indication of how hard you are working. However, during pregnancy there is typically an increased resting heart rate during the early stages of +10–15 beats per minute and a blunted heart rate response towards the end of pregnancy, so just measuring heart rate alone is not accurate enough. Other factors affecting heart rate include how hydrated you are, the time of day, how much sleep you have had, when you last ate and your stress levels. You are better served by using a combination of heart rate—measured by your target heart-rate zone (THRZ), a subjective measurement of how you feel as you exercise, a rate of perceived exertion (RPE) and your breathlessness (via the 'talk test').

Target heart-rate zones (THRZ) for pregnant women

If you did not exercise regularly prior to getting pregnant, then a safe range is 60–70% of your maximum heart rate. If you were active before and want to maintain your fitness throughout your pregnancy, then aim to keep your heart rate between 70–80% of your maximum heart rate. The formula is:

maximum heart rate of 220 _minus_ your age _times_ a percentage intensity

This formula is an average guide only, because there can be quite big differences in maximum heart rate between people of different genetic makeups and fitness levels. Having one maximum heart rate of 220 less an age for the entire population is like having a one-size-fits-all approach. While it is absolutely accurate for about 60% of us, rest assured it is probably only slightly off for the rest. So work yours out now.

(220–your age) x 0.70 = lower training heart-rate figure (beats per minute)

(220–your age) x 0.80 = upper training heart-rate figure (beats per minute)

Your training _range_ is the heart-beat range between the upper and lower figures.

Here is a calculation for a 35-year-old regular exerciser:

(220–35)x0.70=130
(220–35)x0.80=148

Here's a quick-glance chart to help you work out what your training zone should be during pregnancy—bearing in mind that this is just a guide, and that as your pregnancy progresses you will modify and decrease targets accordingly. Note that if you have been doing regular aerobic exercise, your cardiovascular fitness may already be quite good and therefore you may find these targets conservative; if so, work instead from the perceived rate of exertion guide rather than using absolute numbers.

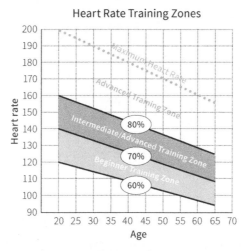

Fig.1.2

Measuring heart rate
Taking your pulse
You can measure heart rate by taking your pulse rate while you are exercising. To do this

you will need a digital watch or one with a second hand. Put your fingertips on the thumb side of your wrist; don't use your thumb as it has its own pulse. Slide your fingers towards the centre of your wrist; you should feel the pulse between the wrist bone and the tendon. Do not press too hard or you will not be able to feel the regular pulsation. If you find timing yourself over a minute too difficult or tedious, try it over 10 seconds taking extra care to count the pulses—then refer to the chart for 10-second target heart-rate zones for your age (Fig.1.3).

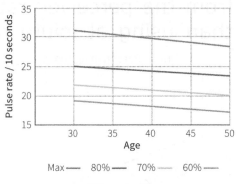

Fig.1.3

Other ways of measuring heart rate

A heart-rate monitor consists of an elasticised chest strap that transmits to a wrist watch. These used to be expensive gadgets for the likes of competitive athletes, but there are many reasonably priced models available now—you will only need a model that has basic functions, like heart-rate measurement and perhaps the ability to set upper and lower limits. Some gym fitness machines may have a heart-rate monitor inbuilt and all you have to do is put your hands on the sensor pads and the electronic display will read your heart rate. Again, remember that measuring your heart rate with any of the above methods is a very general measure, but in combination the two self-checks below (RPE and the talk test) you will quickly be able to gauge the right level of intensity for you.

My handy personal trainer

During my first pregnancy I regularly used a wrist-watch heart-rate monitor. My original watch was over 10 years old, so I upgraded recently and interestingly, like many new mass-marketed technologies, the cost had decreased. I am wary of buying gadgets when it comes to fitness. Case in point: how many of you have abdominal machines (abdominisers) gathering dust in the back shed? But this is one piece of equipment that really delivers and seems to last well, despite being dropped and flung into gym bags. I often say it is like having a personal trainer strapped to your wrist, but without the chaffing. They are usually waterproof, too, so you can wear them in the pool. Other functions offered, like calorie-counting and a stopwatch, are fancy window dressing and not

> *really necessary, but these days are often included with a basic model.*

Rate of perceived exertion (RPE)—how you feel about how hard you are exercising

Dr Gunnar Borg from Stockholm University developed a recognised table, which he named it after himself: Borg's Rate of Perceived Exertion (RPE).

Don't ask me why it starts at 6, it just does. This measure is how you feel when you are in horizontal in bed (i.e., doing nothing), and 20 is how you feel when you are absolutely at your maximum exertion and feeling as if you are about to expire.

15-point scale

6—20% effort: no effort at all; lying down, not moving

7—30% effort: extremely light, virtually at rest

8—40% effort

9—50% effort: very light: gentle slow walking

10—55% effort

11—60% effort: fairly light

12—65% effort

13—70% effort: somewhat hard; steady pace
14—75% effort
15—80% effort: hard
16—85% effort
17—90% effort: very hard
18—95% effort
19—100% effort: very, very hard
20—exhaustion

On this Borg scale, pregnant women should be aiming for an exercise level between 12 and 14. So if someone asked you how hard you were working out, you would reply along the lines of 'somewhat hard'.

10-point scale
Let's make RPE easier to remember by adapting the above table to be an intensity guide ranging between 1 and 10.

1—no effort at all: couch potato
2—extremely light: lifting my glass up
3—very light: walking easily
4—fairly light: can talk OK, starting to heat up
5—above comfortable: somewhat hard, beginning to puff
6—putting in effort: sweating, slightly breathless
7—moderate to hard: conversation limited, panting

8—hard: this is intense, can't continue for too long
9—very hard: ouch, short burst only
10—maximum, exhaustion, no go anymore

Beginner exercisers would want to aim for a level 5 RPE, and build up to an RPE of 6 to 7. Those women previously active should be exercising at around level 6 to 7.

The talk test—another subjective measurement of intensity

When you are not pregnant the 'talk test' works like this: when exercising at the correct intensity you are able to speak 'in sentences of ... *[breath]*.... three or four ... *[breath]*.......... words, but then ... *[breath]*.......... you would have ... *[breath]*.......... to take a breath'. That puffing and panting level is about the right intensity for normal aerobic fat-burning exercise. However, now that you are pregnant you need to decrease the intensity, which means you should be able to comfortably maintain a conversation as you exercise. What? Talk and exercise? Yes, the good news is you no longer need to go to a café to have a chat to your friend; instead, you can go for a health-promoting walk together and still catch up on all the latest gossip! If you are out of breath and unable to natter on—slow down. Pregnancy is a journey, not a race. This 'talk test' method of determining how hard you are exercising applies to all three trimesters.

Adapting intensity levels over time

As your own unique pregnancy progress and symptoms appear, you will need to adapt your intensity levels accordingly.

Going faster and harder

Working out faster and harder than your aerobic target zone results in anaerobic exercise where you are puffing and panting. Anaerobic exercise is when the body is craving oxygen but the high level of exertion means the lungs and blood supply can't keep up with demand. An oxygen deficit results after about 30 to 90 seconds of intense activity and the body then sends a strong message to slow down. This is generally too strenuous for pregnancy.

> *With my second pregnancy at the age of 45, I was advised to be super careful in the first trimester given my history and the IVF efforts we had gone to in order to get a positive pregnancy result. Because of this I*

> *dropped right back on the frequency and intensity of my exercise. In fact, it was mainly just walking for the first few months. As a result, once I felt more confident about the pregnancy progressing through the second trimester, my resumption of exercise was definitely modified and any cardiovascular exercise was totally based on my THRZ.*

Tiredness or laziness?

If you don't feel like exercising on a particular day, then DON'T! You won't get any medals for pushing yourself to the limit or beyond. It's not about that now; it's about caring for your body and nurturing your growing baby. Tuning in and listening to the signals your body provides during pregnancy is vitally important. For women who are over 35, the weariness factor can be quite pronounced, especially if you are working until shortly before the birth.

Tiredness is a normal symptom of being pregnant; after all, your body is busy growing another human being. Feeling tired is most common in the first and third trimesters. So long as it is genuine tiredness and not procrastination or laziness, then take a break. However, if it is one the latter two reasons, then just cast your eye back over the list of benefits of exercising during pregnancy and that should help you get motivated. It is often said that the hardest thing about exercising is putting on your shoes and getting out the door. Once you out, you are into it.

If it is more than tiredness—if you are feeling exhausted and are unable to complete the normal activities you do in a day—then you need to pause and consider what might be the cause. Try to determine whether it is the exercise that is contributing to this sense of exhaustion or another variable in your life: for example, doing long, extra hours at work; an increase in negative stress around you; you have missed a few good nights' sleep; or you have been sick. If you think it is the exercise, then take a few days off and see whether your energy levels return. If they do, then modify what you are attempting. Remember: don't overdo it. While 'if a little is good, then a lot must be better' might apply to some things, it does *not* apply to exercising during pregnancy.

Overtraining, whether you are pregnant or not, can bring about deep-seated tiredness, a lack of interest in exercising, lack of motivation and susceptibility to illness and infection. The signs of overtraining are obvious in the pregnant mother and can also be observed in the fetus. If you are doing too much, the baby's growth rate will slow. Your LMC will be monitoring growth rate, so both of you will be able to note any decrease in normal growth rate and make the necessary steps to decrease your exercising appropriately.

From mid- to late pregnancy the normal course of events is for the baby to move a few times in the 30 minutes following your exercise session. If there is ever a case where you think the movements have slowed markedly, stopped or something just isn't right, then seek advice immediately from your LMC. It doesn't take long to do a scan or measure the baby's heart rate, and it can give you the peace of mind you need.

If you think it is stress that may be causing you to be exhausted, then modify your exercise programme to accommodate that. I wouldn't suggest stopping altogether, as exercise has been shown to be a wonderful antidote to the build-up of negative stress. Exercise and being fit also allow greater relaxation.

All through your pregnancy journey you will need to adjust and modify your fitness goals depending on your overall wellbeing. You are not a machine; you are a holistic being, so the best approach is to proceed with a flexible attitude while being aware of tuning in to your body's needs and signals.

> *Remember: don't overdo it. Sometimes less can be more for pregnant women. Treat your body with the extra respect it deserves at this time in your life.*

Playing sport when pregnant

Attitudes have changed in this millennium as regards the participation of pregnant sportswomen at a competitive level. Some sportswomen have chosen to carry on competing at an élite level well into pregnancy; others have chosen to retire from competitive endeavours once pregnant. It is a personal choice and always should be made in consultation with your LMC. The medical consensus now is that women who have normal pregnancies and who are already active can continue to play many sports during early to mid-pregnancy without affecting the course or outcome of their pregnancy. By late pregnancy it is usually simply not physically possible to perform at such a high level.

Something that sportswomen have to weigh up is an increasing vulnerability to falls due to their changing centre of gravity as their pregnancy progresses, affecting both balance and co-ordination. That said, at a national forum on pregnancy and sport in Australia, the issue was thrashed out, with medical experts agreeing that 'falls and direct contact of the kinds that occur during contact sports were unlikely to cause damage to the womb or the unborn child'. They concluded that 'damage to the womb of the kind that could injure an unborn child is usually associated with forces equivalent to those occurring in a car accident' *(Australian Sports Commission 2002 Report).*

Hormonal changes in mid- to late pregnancy result in the softening of ligaments and corresponding joint laxity, and this may also pose a potential risk of injury. Most sporting codes will advise pregnant athletes that there may be risks involved and to get medical advice on those risks. The pregnant athlete can then decide in consultation with their own medical advisors when to continue playing, when to taper off, and when to cease their involvement.

General advice to athletes

* Obtain expert medical advice.

* Understand the risks, use common sense, and take into account changes in your physical condition.

* Keep intensity at less than 75% of your maximum heart rate.

* Regularly review your training and performance.

* See a doctor immediately if there are any warning signs such as bleeding or abdominal pain.

> *Statistically, getting pregnant in your thirties and forties is a gift, so make sure you don't jeopardise that 'gift' by sticking to rigid sporting routines and pushing yourself hard.*

There will be plenty of years ahead to resume your sporting prowess. Now is a time to go easy on your body and keep just moderately fit so your pregnancy can bloom.

Fitting exercise into a busy life

Even once the benefits of regular exercise are acknowledged, it can be another thing altogether to fit it into an already busy life, particularly when you already have other children. As a mother of two, I do understand the extra effort and planning required to continue exercising when you have children of varying ages nipping at your heels and wanting constant attention. There is no doubt it is a challenge to fit it in, and it sometimes requires Herculean efforts.

For me, and for many active mums, physical exercise and mental relaxation go hand in hand. In fact, actual workout time can sometimes be the only mental switch-off time you have in your day, slotted in around the demands of work, children and fulfilling your share of keeping the household functioning.

I have found the only way I have been able to continue with what I regard as an important healthy component of my lifestyle is to:

√ decide that exercise must be a priority—it has to be otherwise it will always be on the get-around-to list, and that benefits no one

√ plan a week ahead—literally get out your diary and write in what you plan to do

√ utilise the kids club or crèche at your local gym, it can be a lifesaver

√ incorporate some exercise options that have the kids or family involved

√ team up with another mum to babysit or do 'kiddy drop-offs' so each of you can do some exercise.

Chapter 2

Nourish Your Body During Pregnancy

If you are over 35, it's likely you're eating a better diet than you did when you were in your twenties. However, pregnancy is the most nutritionally demanding time of a woman's life, so it is never too late to start eating well.

The importance of nutrition

✳ Good nutrition affects the future health outcomes of your unborn child.

✳ Good nutrition makes your journey through pregnancy easier and more enjoyable.

✳ Good nutrition during pregnancy affects your future health and wellbeing.

What you consume, directly and quickly affects your growing baby through maternal blood being passed to the fetus through the placenta and umbilicus. Ensuring what you eat is balanced and nutritious means you are giving your unborn child the best possible chance of developing in the womb. If you are looking after your body in every other way, then it follows that naturally you are going to want to be sensible about what you eat and drink.

Babies born to mothers who have had poor nutrition during pregnancy can exhibit learning difficulties, reduced growth, dental problems, allergies, and be more prone to illness.

Weight gain

A burning question from many newly pregnant women is how much weight should they put on. The answer depends on how much you weighed pre-conception and how that relates to your body mass index (BMI), which indicates total body dimension.

Body mass index

To calculate your BMI, divide your weight in kilograms by your height in metres squared. For example, if you are 1.65 metres tall and weigh 64 kilograms, your BMI is calculated as follows:

$$BMI = \frac{weight}{height^2} \quad \frac{kg}{m^2}$$

$$BMI = \frac{64}{1.65^2 \atop (1.65 \times 1.65)} \quad \frac{64}{2.7225} = 23.5$$

Now calculate your own BMI.

My weight = _____ kg

My height = _____ m

$$\text{My BMI} = \frac{\text{kg}}{\text{m}^2} =$$

Use the range below to see what your BMI means in terms of your health.

 ❋ A BMI of less than 20 means you are underweight.

 ❋ A BMI between 20 and 25 means your weight is normal.

 ❋ A BMI between 26 and 30 means you are overweight.

 ❋ A BMI over 30 means you are obese.

Effect of BMI on pregnancy weight gain

Have a look at this chart and plot where your pre-pregnancy weight sits in relation to your height. Note, however, that there are limitations to this formula, as it does not differentiate between fat and muscle, and muscle is heavier than fat. Healthy weight ranges also differ depending on a person's ethnicity. For example, European and Maori women will have a healthy BMI sitting somewhere between 20 and 25. Pasifika women will naturally be slightly higher, and Asian women slightly lower, so take this as a general guide only.

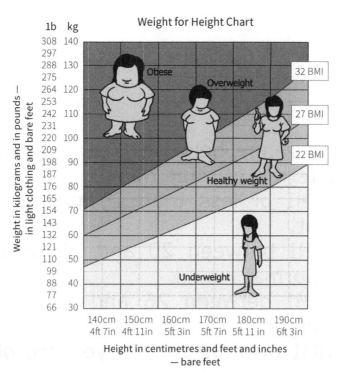

Fig.2.1

All women should expect to gain weight during pregnancy, especially in the second and third trimesters. If your pre-pregnancy weight was in the healthy range for your height (a BMI of 20 to 25), you should gain 11.5–16 kilograms, gaining 0.5–2.5 kilograms in the first trimester, and about 0.5 kilograms per week for the rest of your pregnancy for the optimal growth of your baby.

If you were **underweight** for your height at conception (a BMI below 18.5), you should gain around 12–18 kilograms, and make sure to increase your consumption of protein and high-energy foods.

If you were **significantly overweight** for your height (a BMI of close to or more than 30), you should gain 6–8 kilograms. It is not a time to diet, so forget quantity and instead concentrate on quality by making sure you consume adequate protein, vitamins and minerals.

If you are having **a multiple pregnancy,** this will increase your nutritional demands, particularly folic acid and iron, so ask your LMC if you require a supplement.

'Eating for two'

For some women, falling pregnant is like gaining a permission slip to eat with reckless abandon and damn the calories. Unfortunately, when you give birth it is just to a baby and not to all those excess calories you have consumed under the misconception that you needed to eat for two.

The actual amount of extra calories required daily to sustain a pregnancy is only about 300. Here is an idea of what that equates to.

Healthy food choices equating to approximately 300 calories:

√ 1 cup of non-fat fruit yogurt and a medium apple

√ 1 piece of wholegrain toast spread with 2 tablespoons peanut butter

√ 1 cup of raisin bran cereal with 1/2 cup of non-fat milk and a small banana

√ 1 flour tortilla (7-inch), 1/2 cup refried beans, 1/2 cup cooked broccoli, and 1/2 cup cooked red pepper.

So sadly it is not extra servings every day, and it is not lashings of cream on top of pudding every night.

And consider this: if you overeat during pregnancy, you are making the job of getting back into shape following the birth that much harder. Do you really want to give yourself a Mount Everest to climb, or would you rather practise some moderation now? A taste of a treat can often satisfy that burning desire for sugar or fatty foods—so have the taste, just don't consume the lot.

Pregnancy is not the time to over-eat or under-eat. It is certainly not the time to try to lose weight or diet; nor is it the time to pig out. The physical consequences of such over-consumption during pregnancy will not magically melt away. It will require solid hard work exercising and modifying your diet after giving birth, and let's face it, by then you will have a precious little baby competing for your time. Excess weight gain will also make you more prone to gestational diabetes. Make your life easier by making the choice now to manage a healthy and sensible weight gain during your pregnancy.

Note that other dietary considerations need to be made during pregnancy to ensure the optimum mix of food groups in your diet. These are discussed below, under 'Essentials'. Note, too, that people with different dietary requirements or lifestyles, such as being vegetarian, may need to take specific steps to ensure the right balance or uptake of nutrients; again, this is discussed under 'Essentials'.

Attitude to food

Your attitude to food during pregnancy should be, whenever possible, to eat nourishing, wholesome food. Your body is undergoing enormous change and adaptation to grow a whole new being, so give it the best help you can by providing healthy nutritious food sources.

There are three key words to keep forefront of mind when making healthy food choices during pregnancy and beyond: balance, variety and moderation.

✳ **Balance** Enjoy a good balance between the various food groups. Try to avoid bingeing on one type of food or excluding others.

✳ **Variety** Eat with the seasons, experimenting with fresh fruit and vegetables to create variety. Try to avoid getting into boring habits and cooking the same old meals every night. Explore new cooking styles, foods you haven't tried before, and keep an eye out for low-fat options. (But bear in mind the foods you should avoid in pregnancy, as discussed below.) Research shows that the greater the variety in your diet, the better your health will be.

   ✳   **Moderation** Forget forbidden food lists—they just set you up for failure. And forget dieting as it is a sure way to ensure you will pack the weight back on. Practise moderation, especially at parties, restaurants, takeaway bars, and other places where the healthy food choices may be limited.

Blood sugar and eating little and often

One of the most important practices in a healthy diet is not skipping meals, as your body needs a regular supply of nutrients and water. This is even more important in pregnancy, as you are supporting the development and growth of another human being. As soon as you go without food for longer than four to five hours, your blood sugar or energy levels run low. Research shows that during pregnancy the body channels even more blood sugar to the growing fetus and less to mum, so blood sugar lows or drops can be quite quick and marked unless you eat in a manner to counteract this effect.

You may not be in the habit of snacking between meals, but during pregnancy this is definitely something to consider. Not everyone has to, but it pays to be prepared. Have emergency snack packs of food in your car, at work or in your handbag so you can avoid going for long periods without food. The way you space out your food intake over the day depends on your lifestyle, job, exercise habits and what you are currently used to. In general, pregnant women do better with smaller, more frequent food intakes. You may even want to try the grazing approach—six small meals over the day. If you are a grazer, remember it is not a case of having six full meals, rather it is taking the approximate content of three normal meals and splitting it over six mini-meals. The grazing approach does require forward thinking and planning so that you have the right sort of food on hand to eat—especially if you are out and about.

During my first pregnancy my relationship with food was the opposite to what I was expecting. I lost my appetite. In fact, in my first trimester I lost weight—something I was certainly not attempting to do. However, it wasn't a dramatic loss, thankfully, just enough for me to notice a looser fit and feel of my clothes. It all worked out in the end, though, with my pregnancy weight gain being in the normal range. I stacked it on where and when it mattered—growing a good 3410-gram baby

(7 pound 5 ounces), and despite that initial lack of appetite I still had to put in the effort and exercise to get my pre-pregnancy body back!

During my second pregnancy I had sustained morning sickness that lasted most of the day, a suppressed appetite and a nightly craving for chocolate Paddle Pops (a milk-based ice-block). In the third trimester I had lots of indigestion which was alleviated by over-the-counter, pregnancy-safe antacids.

Some healthy snack ideas

✓ Fruit—fresh or pottles of fruit
✓ Yoghurt
✓ Milk-based drinks, smoothies
✓ Crackers with a topping—cheese, hummus, tomato, vegemite, avocado, etc.
✓ Vegetable sticks
✓ Fruit cake, fruit muffins, bran muffins
✓ Toast
✓ Sandwiches, cheese on toast
✓ Nuts and dried fruit

Must-haves during pregnancy

Below is a checklist of some of the essentials for your diet for a healthy pregnancy. These are discussed more fully later in the chapter.

✓ Some extra calories—around 300 per day, preferably in the form of carbohydrates (energy suppliers)

✓ Protein—extra supplies

✓ Fluid—at least 6–8 cups per day, more if you are exercising or in a warm climate

✓ Iron—you need twice as much when you are pregnant than when you aren't—about 27 milligrams each day

✓ Folic acid—minimum of 600 micrograms of folic acid a day (it is common for prenatal supplements to contain 800 micrograms)

✓ Vitamins B, C and D

✓ Calcium—you need about 1200–1300 milligrams each day to make sure both you and your baby get sufficient

✓ Zinc and magnesium

Things to avoid or minimise

Foods to avoid

Due to food bacteria posing a threat to your baby, it is important to be extra vigilant when it comes to food safety, hygiene and food choices. The common food bacteria *Listeria* can survive and multiply in the fridge. Avoid the following foods while you are pregnant as they have a high risk of contamination:

✕ raw eggs (often used in mayonnaise, smoothies, etc.)

✕ raw and smoked animal foods; shellfish, raw fish, smoked fish

✕ sushi—all types (the rice can be a problem as well as the filling)

✕ cold pre-cooked chicken, ham and all other chilled pre-cooked meat products, rare cooked meat

✕ pâté, pre-prepared salads, hummus

✕ soft unpasteurised cheese, such as Roquefort

✕ soft-serve ice cream

✕ cold leftovers.

Heat can eliminate some of the bacterial risk, so some foods can be consumed if they have been cooked thoroughly and are steaming hot—but if in doubt, leave it out. To make sure your chilled food is really cold, get a temperature gauge from the hardware store and check that your fridge is tuned to 1–5° Celsius.

Check the 'best before' and 'use by' dates on packages before buying or consuming. If it doubt, throw it out.

For a comprehensive list of foods to avoid, food safety guidelines, tips on eating out, and food issues to be aware of when travelling, check your government health department website.

Chemical exposure

The placenta protects the baby to some extent from toxic substances, but it can't block things out completely. Artificial substances and products that you choose to use or consume may be tolerable by you as an adult, but may *not* be tolerated well by your growing baby. There is much discussion but no definitive research to say exposure to normal household chemicals or food additives definitively affects the fetus, but then again there is none that says it definitely doesn't. It is totally up to you how fastidious you are in avoiding exposure to chemicals during this time, but I would suggest a moderate and considered approach: if you are able to avoid them without too much hassle, then do so.

In terms of what you ingest, minimise your consumption of artificial flavours and food dyes. This won't be hard if you are opting for wholesome, nutritious food choices during your pregnancy. Cut down or eliminate nitrates which are contained in highly processed meat products (for example, luncheon sausage and hot dogs). Nitrosamines formed from nitrates have been shown in animal studies to produce cancer in test subject offspring. Good levels of vitamin C in the body can block nitrosamine formation.

In terms of skin absorption or inhalation of chemicals, wherever possible try to remove yourself from environments where chemicals might be found—new paint drying, garden weed spraying, smoky environments. Use rubber gloves with household cleaners to avoid absorbing trace amounts of chemicals through your skin, and if the oven has to be cleaned, you have my permission *for at least this nine months* to get someone else to do it!

I have also heard of women choosing not to get their hair dyed, not using fake tan and ditching the makeup. It is a totally personal choice as to the level you change your lifestyle in order to avoid chemicals, but if you keep in mind that your baby is vulnerable and unable to make the choice themselves I'm sure you will err on the side of 'natural and wholesome' rather than 'overly processed and artificial'.

Alcohol

Research concludes there is no safe limit for alcohol during pregnancy. So the best advice is to avoid it completely for the sake of your baby. In the past the message was less clear, with varying amounts tolerated in different countries. However, now the widespread, definitive message is to avoid any alcohol in order to prevent fetal alcohol spectrum disorder (FASD), which results in intellectual impairment of the baby.

Absolute no-nos

✕ **Smoking** may increase the risk of miscarriage and deprives your developing baby of oxygen and nutrients.

✕ **Drugs and medications** of any kind unless specifically under the monitoring and guidance of your LMC/doctor.

Hydration

About 50–70% of our body weight consists of water and we can only survive for a few days without it. In a pregnancy with normal weight gain, about 3–3.5 kilograms of that is water. Dehydration is the unpleasant side-effect of a lack of water and can result in muscle cramps, dizziness, headaches, fainting, nausea and vomiting.

Try to remember to drink before you get thirsty, because thirst is an indicator that you are already dehydrated. A good habit to get into is to have a glass of water every time you have a meal or a snack. Regardless of being pregnant, ideally you should guzzle around eight glasses a day and even more when you exercise—both before and after the activity. Most of us don't and so are chronically dehydrated. There is of course a very quick fix: drink more water. Specifically, pregnant mothers should have a water-bottle handy so they can take regular sips and keep hydrated throughout the day. Another warning sign of dehydration is bright yellow, pungent urine. If you keep yourself hydrated, your urine should be a pale straw colour. You will also be amazed how much better you feel.

You will no doubt find you are taking more trips to the toilet, especially in the first and last trimesters—so being told to drink up might sound to you like a prison sentence of spending even more time in the bathroom. However this is just one of those frustrating symptoms of being pregnant and one you will need to tolerate.

Don't get dehydrated, for your baby's sake. Allowing yourself to get dehydrated can subject the baby to the unwanted side-effect of increased temperature in the womb—remember, the baby is always hotter than you are. Dehydration can cause your circulation to become sluggish and that affects blood flow and nutrition to the baby. Dehydration can also make you more susceptible to urine infections. So get drinking. The best fluids to drink are water, diluted fruit juice, or low-fat milk. You could spice up your water with a slice of lemon or cucumber, some mint leaves, ice cubes, or a drop of lime—anything to make you drink more.

Monitoring water intake

If you are unsure as to how much water you are drinking on a daily basis, get yourself a 2-litre plastic bottle, fill it with water and see if you get through its entire contents over the course of one day. A glass of water is approximately 250 millilitres, so eight of them equals 2 litres. You may be shocked at how little you are actually drinking.

Good tips for increasing water consumption

✓ Drink a glass of water first thing in the morning

✓ Every time you have a drink of tea or coffee, have a glass of water too

✓ Drink before, during and after exercising

✓ Get into the habit of having a glass of water with every meal

✓ Keep water bottles in your handbag and car. Fill them regularly and sip, sip, sip.

Fluids—but not thirst-quenchers

Concentrated fruit juices actually require dilution by the body for digestion, which means the body seeks out water from your tissues. They also contain a lot of sugar, so get into the habit of diluting pure juices with water by half.

Tea and coffee are liquids, but they have a mild diuretic action due to their caffeine content; that means they cause the body to eliminate water.

Most soft drinks (except the diet or low cal versions) have a high sugar content and again require the body to seek out water from elsewhere in the body to dilute them for digestion. Some also have caffeine in them, so be aware of product contents.

Minimise or eliminate consumption of caffeine

Caffeine acts as a stimulant to the heart and central nervous system, and is also known to increase blood pressure in the short term, although there is no conclusive evidence of long-term effects on blood pressure.

Caffeine content of some drinks

Average caffeine content	Serving size	Caffeine (mg)
Long black – café*	160ml	211
Decaf long black coffee	130ml	19
Cappuccino – café*	260ml	105
Instant coffee*	250ml	51
Plunger coffee*	250ml	66
Tea made with tea bag*	250ml	47
Brewed tea leaves*	250ml	57
Drinking chocolate/cocoa*	250ml	15
Smart or energy drinks	250ml	80
Cola-type drinks	355ml	35

Average caffeine content	Serving size	Caffeine (mg)
Chocolate bar	100g	65

* Figures may alter depending on strength and method of making

As caffeine travels through the placenta, high doses are not good for your baby. Research concludes that consumption of caffeine is best minimised or avoided altogether by pregnant women, with the current recommendation for no more than 300mg of caffeine to be consumed per day.

For an avid coffee-lover like myself this poses something of a challenge, so during my pregnancy I got decaffeinated beans for grinding at home and always asked for decaf when out and about.

Remember tea also contains caffeine, as do energy drinks.

Essentials

Carbohydrate

Carbohydrate is the best fuel for the body's engine. The human body converts carbohydrate to glucose, which the cells use for energy. Any glucose that you don't need immediately is transformed into glycogen and stored in the liver and muscles where it is kept as an energy reserve. If this isn't used up, it is eventually—and inefficiently—stored as fat.

Carbohydrates come in two forms:

* **simple carbohydrates**—sugars such as honey and jam
* **complex carbohydrates**—from cereals, rice, pasta, bread, fruit and vegetables

Foods rich in complex carbohydrates are a better energy source than simple sugars, because they are rich in other nutrients such as fibre, protein, vitamins and minerals, and they are converted more slowly, which means they will keep your energy levels high longer. Simple carbohydrates tend to be absorbed quickly and can rapidly increase the sugar levels in your blood, which is then followed a short time later by a 'crash' or drop in blood sugar.

Carbohydrates currently make up about 46% of average daily food intake. Ideally, they should supply at least half of our daily energy intake, and preferably be around 55–60%.

Good sources of carbohydrate are wholemeal bread, pita pockets, fruit bread, wholemeal rice, fruit and root vegetables, rice cakes, rice, pasta, dried beans and lentils, porridge, yogurt and milk.

Carbohydrates and pregnancy

In the first trimester your body will use more carbohydrates, and this can result in you feeling tired and less energetic than normal. You should find this is relieved somewhat in the second trimester, and by the third trimester, when the baby is utilising more proteins than carbohydrates for growth, you should have your energy zing back. However, bear in mind that by that stage other factors will probably slow you down a little, like your increased weight and size.

Protein

Proteins are made of smaller components called amino acids. There are 23 amino acids, of which eight are termed essential amino acids—these can't be made by your body and must be supplied from what you consume. Protein is a vital part of every cell in the body, including those in the muscles, heart, liver, kidneys, blood cells, skin, hair, nails, teeth and bones. It is essential for growth, and for the repair and formation of new cells, hence its crucial role during pregnancy. Protein is vital for fighting infection, too, because it helps make antibodies, and it also helps produce haemoglobin, which carries oxygen through the bloodstream, and hormones, such as insulin.

Dieticians recommend that 12–15% of the energy intake in a healthy daily diet comes from protein. Unfortunately, many of us eat more than twice this, and get protein from high-fat foods, such as hamburger patties, and fatty meat like bacon and sausages. The healthy option is to choose lean protein sources, like meat that is red without lots of accompanying white fat alongside. The right combination of vegetable protein foods can also supply all the necessary amino acids.

Protein is not the body's preferred first energy source to utilise during exercise; it is well down the list. This is because protein is only burned as an energy source during starvation, extreme dieting or when we eat far more protein than we actually need.

During pregnancy you need a slight increase in protein above the normal daily requirements of 0.2 grams per kilogram of body weight. During breastfeeding you need a little more again—1.1 grams per kilogram of body weight. So let's say you weigh 65 kilograms, that means an extra 13 grams of protein a day during pregnancy which you could get from one pot of low-fat yogurt and a glass of milk, or a chicken drumstick (skin removed) or two eggs, or a handful of almonds.

Good sources of protein during pregnancy include trim milk, yogurt, low-fat cheese, eggs (cooked), lean meat, chicken (no skin), fish (tinned or fresh), nuts, dried beans and lentils, tinned beans, chickpeas or soup mix. Women who are vegetarian can find good protein sources in legumes (such as baked beans, lentils, chickpeas, soya beans), nuts, dairy products (cheese, milk) and, to a lesser extent, a range of vegetables and cereals (pasta, muesli, wholemeal bread). You may also wish to consider easing up on strict vegetarianism for the duration of your pregnancy to ensure both you and your baby get adequate protein, and in particular an essential mineral that comes from meat-based protein—iron. If that is not an option, seek advice from your LMC about changes you can make to the way you eat (for example, tea restricts iron uptake, so do not drink tea with meals). Organisations like the Vegetarian Society have helpful material on adjusting diet during pregnancy. Iron absorption is discussed in more detail later in the chapter, under 'Iron'.

Fat

We need some fat in our diet ... just not the amount that we actually consume. Fat is the biggest downfall of the Western diet. We eat too much of the stuff: it accounts for about 40% of the typical daily energy intake. If we reduce our fat proportion to about 30%, we reduce our risk from a whole raft of illnesses, such as heart disease, high blood pressure, obesity, diabetes, gallstones and some types of cancers.

Scientists refer to fats as 'lipids'. They come in both animal and vegetable foods and they make food taste good, which is why most of us like fat with our meals. Unfortunately, fats contain more than twice as many kilojoules as proteins or carbohydrates, so it is easy to overdo your intake. The result: your body stores the excess and you start packing on the fat.

There are two main types of fat: saturated and unsaturated. Most fatty foods contain a mixture of both. **Saturated fats** are found in fatty meats, some dairy products and chocolate. Saturated fats are bad news for heart health. They contribute to 'bad' cholesterol and reduce levels of 'good' cholesterol, putting you more at risk of heart disease and some cancers, including bowel cancer. Coconut oil is a saturated fat but has received recent good press after being touted as a super-food. However, regardless of whatever other benefits it may or may not offer, it is still a saturated fat. Perhaps its current positive profile is because coconut oil is made up of medium-chain fatty acids which are considered heart-friendlier than the long-chain counterparts found in animal products.

Polyunsaturated fats, such as those found in margarine and vegetable oils, are somewhat more desirable. They have been found to reduce levels of 'good' cholesterol in the blood, but they reduce 'bad' cholesterol even more, and they supply essential fatty acids which the body needs but can't make. However, they have been linked with some cancers, especially breast cancer.

Monounsaturated fats are found in olive oil, avocados, canola and linseed oil, peanuts and peanut oils as well as oily fish. They are the best kind of fats you can eat as they raise good cholesterol and reduce bad cholesterol. Communities which have a high intake of monounsaturated fats tend to have lower rates of breast cancer, but scientists don't yet know if that's because these fats protect them or because of their low dietary intake of saturated fat, or because of some other aspect of their diet.

French and Mediterranean people have a considerably lower incidence of heart disease than Australasians, despite their high-fat diet which includes cheese, olives, olive oil and avocados. The secret might be in the type of fat they consume. The average Mediterranean diet contains more vegetable-based fats (monosaturated) and less animal fats (saturated) than our diet, and these factors contribute to the healthy difference.

Important fats during pregnancy

Of particular importance are omega 3 fats which are found in oily fish such as salmon and tuna, as they promote healthy fetal development. Omega 3 fats are required by every cell in the body. Researchers have found that omega 3 supplementation during pregnancy may improve the child's hand-and-eye co-ordination. However, a warning: pregnant women should not eat certain kinds of deep-sea or long-living fish, because they may contain high levels of a form of mercury that can be harmful to the developing fetus. This means avoid eating shark, swordfish, king mackerel, marlin, and so on, during your pregnancy. Albacore tuna is high in mercury, too, so you may want to choose canned tuna instead. Other types of fish are fine in limited amounts; for example, about two fish meals per week. Don't ditch the fish completely because of the warning above, just choose the right sort of fish. Get the benefits of a good source of protein, omega 3 fats and other nutrients that fish as a food source provides.

Vitamins important for pregnancy

Folic acid (also called folate, folacin, and vitamin B^9)

Folic acid is a vitamin which women require at boosted levels during pregnancy to assist with development of the nervous system of the baby. Low levels are associated with neural tube defects—spina bifida and anencephaly, which are caused by incomplete development of the brain, the spinal cord or their protective coverings in early pregnancy. It is well researched that increasing the amount of folic acid in your diet prior to getting pregnant and in the first trimester can prevent birth defects such as deformities, brain damage, spina bifida or other complications like a premature birth or a low-weight baby.

Supplementation

The recommended dietary intake (RDI) for adults is 400 micrograms per day, and this increases to 600 micrograms per day for women who are planning to become pregnant or are in the first trimester of pregnancy. In New Zealand, it is recommended that women should take one 800 micrograms (0.8 milligrams) folic acid tablet daily for at least 4 weeks before and 12 weeks after conception (the first trimester) as well as consuming foods rich in folate and folic acid fortified foods. In Australia, from late 2009 it became law that all bread (except organic) must have added folic acid. The mandatory additive is a relatively small amount, so women intending to fall pregnant are still encouraged to take folic acid supplements well before they start trying to conceive. However, this new law fortifying bread will provide a benefit for unplanned pregnancies and brings Australia into line with other Western countries, including the United States and Canada. New Zealand has retained a voluntary code for bread manufacturers.

Its role

Folic acid is important in the formation of new body cells, particularly red blood cells, and in the transmission of information from genes to cells. It is also critical for DNA synthesis and cell growth, energy production and forming amino acids.

Effects of having too little
Having too little folic acid can lead to fetal neural tube defects (see above), anaemia (common in pregnant women worldwide) and reduced endurance.

Effects of having too much
Large doses may disguise a vitamin B_{12} deficiency.

Food sources
Folic acid can be found in broccoli, avocados, green leafy vegetables (wash well before use), legumes, citrus fruits, yeast extract, wholegrain breads, and liver (but limit intake to 100 grams per week due to the high vitamin A levels in liver; it needs to be well cooked, served hot, and eaten immediately after cooking).

Vitamin A (retinol)—avoid extra amounts
Pregnant women should not take excess vitamin A, as it is toxic to the fetus and can produce severe congenital deformities. Pregnant women should not take supplements containing vitamin A; however, a normal varied diet will not cause an oversupply of vitamin A.

Its role

Vitamin A is important for vision, growth, reproduction, fighting infection and keeping the skin and gut healthy.

Effects of having too little

Prolonged deficiency can cause blindness, stunted growth, reduced immunity to infections, dry skin and hair, and night blindness.

Effects of having too much

Excess vitamin A is toxic, causing red, dry skin, irritability, fatigue, loss of appetite, loss of hair, haemorrhages, joint pains, vomiting and possibly even liver damage.

Food sources

Vitamin A can be found in cooked spinach, broccoli, milk, yogurt, liver, fatty fish, and brightly coloured vegetables.

Vitamin D

Vitamin D is essential in pregnancy for the formation of the bones of the baby, and for maintenance of the mother's bone density.

Its role

Vitamin D helps in the absorption of calcium and phosphate, resulting in strong bones and teeth.

Effects of having too little

Vitamin D deficiency leads to a risk of rickets. In adults, especially pregnant women, there is a risk of osteomalacia, which is the softening and bending of bones.

Effects of having too much

Be careful with vitamin D supplements—it's easy to overdose, causing your body to absorb too much calcium, which is deposited in soft tissues such as the spleen and kidneys. Symptoms include vomiting, loss of appetite, weakness, and irritability.

Food sources

Most vitamin D is produced in the body from the action of ultraviolet light from the sun, so get some but not too many of the sun's rays. Food sources are fish liver oil, tuna, salmon, and egg yolk. Margarine and dairy products also contain vitamin D.

The B vitamins

This group of vitamins are important during pregnancy as they help release energy during metabolism. They are water-soluble, so any excess is excreted in your urine, often turning it bright yellow.

Vitamin B^1 (thiamin)

Its role

Vitamin B_1 releases energy from carbohydrates, and so is important for the growth and function of the digestive and nervous systems, and the heart. The recommended dietary intake for women is 1.1 milligrams.

Effects of having too little

Deficiency in vitamin B_1 is rare in Western societies except among alcoholics, but it causes muscle weakness and loss of limb function, memory and appetite.

Effects of having too much

Vitamin B_1 is non-toxic.

Food sources

Vitamin B_1 can be found in pork, nuts, wholegrain cereals and breads, brown rice, pasta, fish, and eggs.

Vitamin B^2 (riboflavin)

Its role

Vitamin B_2 is important in the use of protein, and is helpful in the growth and repair of tissues. The recommended dietary intake for women is 1.1 milligrams.

Effects of having too little

Vitamin B_2 deficiency results in cracks at the corners of the mouth and on the lips, shiny, sore red tongue and dermatitis in the creases around the nose. It may cause lowered resistance to infection, and possible increased risk of certain cancers.

Effects of having too much

Excess riboflavin is excreted in the urine.

Food sources

Vitamin B_2 can be found in brewer's yeast, liver, kidney, dairy products, fish, meat, almonds and yeast extract.

Vitamin B^6

Its role

Vitamin B_6 is essential in the activities of certain hormones and enzymes involved in breaking down food, manufacturing red blood cells and antibodies, and in the functioning of the nervous and digestive systems. The recommended dietary intake for women 1.3–1.5 milligrams.

Effects of having too little

Vitamin B_6 deficiency causes weakness, depression, skin disorders, irritability, inflammation of the mouth and tongue, cracked lips, anaemia and seizures (in young children).

Effects of having too much

Massive doses (100 times the recommended daily intake) can cause nerve inflammation.

Food sources

Vitamin B_6 can be found in lentils, beans, fish, bananas, pork, meat, poultry, nuts, potatoes and avocados.

Vitamin B^12

Its role

Vitamin B_{12} is important for the operation of the nervous system and for red blood cell development. Its functions are closely linked with folic acid.

Effects of having too little

Vitamin B_{12} can result in pernicious anaemia, nerve damage, and paralysis.

Effects of having too much

No known effects.

Food sources

Vitamin B_{12} is found in chicken, beef, pork, kidney, liver, fish, eggs, milk, cheese and enriched cereals.

Vitamin C

During pregnancy vitamin C is crucial for maintaining healthy muscles, connective tissue and bones, as well as forming iron from haemoglobin and red blood cells. The recommended dietary intake for women is 45 milligrams.

Its role

Vitamin C is needed to form collagen, which is structural scaffolding for blood vessels, bones, teeth, gums, tendons, and cartilage. It helps produce some proteins and hormones, helps absorb iron, prevents infection, and may reduce blood cholesterol levels. Its antioxidant properties may also help the body's immune system and help prevent cancer.

Effects of having too little

Too little vitamin C reduces resistance to infection and can cause weakness, poor wound healing, and bleeding gums. Prolonged deficiency results in scurvy.

Effects of having too much

Massive doses can cause diarrhoea, kidney stones, and even rebound scurvy; it may also interfere with the effects of drugs like aspirin, antidepressants, anticoagulants and the contraceptive pill.

Food sources

Vitamin C is found in fruit, vegetables and liver. Particularly rich sources include parsley, citrus fruit, capsicum, tomato, strawberries, kiwifruit, broccoli and cabbage.

Vitamin E

Its role

This antioxidant prevents damage to cells from oxygen. It is essential for the formation of haemoglobin and provides protection against toxic chemicals.

Effect of having too little

Vitamin E deficiency leads to the premature destruction of red blood cells in newborn babies, and reduced resistance to tissue oxidation. Deficiency is rare as the body stores considerable amounts of vitamin E.

Effects of having too much

Large doses can cause stomach upsets but are not considered toxic.

Food sources

Vitamin E is found in plants, especially seeds, seed oil, nuts and asparagus, seafood, whole grains, butter and eggs.

Vitamin K

Its role

Vitamin K is essential for forming blood clots.

Effects of having too little

Vitamin K deficiency can result in excessive bleeding and haemorrhages. Babies are particularly at risk until they are old enough to start producing their own supplies, which is why you will be asked whether you will give consent to a vitamin K injection shortly after birth.

Effects of having too much

Few toxic effects are known, but it can cause anaemia.

Food sources

Vitamin K is found in leafy green vegetables, pork, oats and liver. Intestinal bacteria also produce vitamin K, but not enough for our needs.

Minerals important for pregnancy

Calcium—an essential nutrient in pregnancy

Calcium is important for the bone strength and development of both mother and baby. Generally, the calcium requirements of the baby during pregnancy are met through the mother absorbing and retaining more calcium during this time. Calcium also works with vitamin D during pregnancy to reduce pain perception.

Its role

Calcium is pivotal in building strong bones and teeth, and is also needed to help the nervous system, heart and muscles work effectively.

Effects of having too little
Calcium deficiency can lead to porous, fragile bones and the risk of osteoporosis (brittle bone disease).

Effects of having too much
Excessive dietary calcium can cause kidney stones in susceptible people, but most people excrete any excess. For women aged over 19 years, calcium needs are the same when pregnant as when they are not pregnant, as calcium is absorbed and retained more efficiently during pregnancy, so aim for about three servings of dairy foods each day. For example, one serving of dairy food equates to one glass of milk, or one pottle of yoghurt, or 200 grams of cottage cheese or ricotta, or two slices of hard cheese.

Amount of calcium needed per day

Adults	1000 milligrams
Older women (54+)	1300 milligrams
Pregnant women	1000 milligrams, under 19 years increase to 1300 milligrams
Breastfeeding women	1000 milligrams, under 19 years increase to 1300 milligrams

Food sources
High calcium sources include dairy products, such as milk, cheese, cottage cheese, yogurt, ice cream, and custard. Also salmon, shrimps,

tofu, sardines, mussels, fortified soy milk. Medium calcium sources include whole cereals like muesli, green veggies, beans, and nuts. Sources low in calcium include eggs, fruit, butter, fats and oils, pasta, rice, cream, and potato.

Examples of good daily sources of calcium

1 glass of homogenised milk (200 millilitres)	200 milligrams calcium
1 glass of non-fat milk (200 millilitres)	300 milligrams calcium
1 pottle of yogurt (150 grams)	200 milligrams calcium
3 slices of cheddar cheese (40 grams)	300 milligrams calcium
1 cup of ice cream (140 grams)	200 milligrams calcium
1/2 can of sardines (50 grams)	300 milligrams calcium
1 cup of salmon (240 grams)	200 milligrams calcium
1 medium bowl of muesli (80 grams)	200 milligrams calcium
3 (2.5 centimetres) cubes of tofu (125 grams)	200 milligrams calcium
1 cup of cooked broccoli	100 milligrams calcium
1/2 cup of almonds	300 milligrams calcium
1 cup of baked beans (270 grams)	100 milligrams calcium
1/2 cup of dried figs (105 grams)	300 milligrams calcium

If you do not eat dairy products, other rich sources include:
   √ calcium fortified soy milk

✓ canned fish with bones
✓ nuts
✓ green leafy vegetables
✓ dried fruit
✓ tofu
✓ wholegrain breads and cereals.

Calcium for all women

Eating calcium-rich foods should be a priority for every woman who wants to avoid osteoporosis. It is anticipated that one in four women over the age of 60 will break a bone due to osteoporosis, and that is a conservative estimate. Building bone strength is a lifelong health investment everyone should make. The best sources of calcium are listed in the table on this page. Dairy products, including cheese, yogurt and milk, provide the majority of calcium in the average diet. For a healthy approach, choose low-fat, high-calcium options. For an adequate calcium intake your body needs the equivalent of three servings of dairy products a day. If you think your calcium intake is low, then don't wait until tomorrow—do something about it today.

Iron—an essential nutrient during pregnancy
Its role

During pregnancy iron gives protection against anaemia and helps the body manufacture all the extra red blood cells you and your baby need. Iron is vital in keeping your blood and immune system healthy. Iron requirements at least double in pregnancy from the normal recommended dietary intake for women of 18mg to 30–60 milligrams per day, but iron absorption by the body is a relatively difficult process. Estimates suggest that only about 10–20% of the iron consumed is actually absorbed, hence the need for dramatically increased levels of 100 milligrams or more per day to satisfy the necessary building of blood cells in the mother and fetus. Iron requirements are even higher in the third trimester, when the baby starts to lay down its own important stores of iron.

It is hard to get the amount of iron you need from food alone, so most pregnant women take an iron supplement. An unfortunate side-effect is that iron supplements can often cause constipation. To help alleviate this, make sure you drink sufficient fluids, including orange juice to help iron absorption. Prunes or kiwifruit may also provide some relief. Your doctor will also give you information on how to take iron tablets as they are generally better absorbed on an empty stomach. Taking vitamin C at the same time, either in food or supplement form, can assist with iron uptake by the body, but this is the only vitamin you should be taking at the same time as your iron. Vitamins and minerals in a combination tablet can also hinder iron absorption. Caffeine (contained in both in tea and coffee) or milk also hinders absorption, so avoid those around the time of taking your tablet. Your iron level should be monitored throughout your pregnancy by your LMC and this is usually checked at around 12 weeks and at 32–34 weeks.

Effects of having too much

In normal people, excess iron is not absorbed. In people who are genetically at risk, excess iron can cause haemochromatosis, with liver damage, cirrhosis, diabetes and abnormal skin pigmentation.

Food sources of dietary iron—two types

Iron from **animal-sourced foods** is called 'haem iron'. This is iron that comes from red meat, chicken or fish, and is easily absorbed and utilised by the body. A rule of thumb: the redder the meat, the higher the iron content. The best sources include:

✓ beef, kidney and liver (although limit liver intake to 100 grams per week, because of the high vitamin A levels, and ensure that it is well cooked, served hot and eaten immediately after cooking)

✓ veal

✓ lamb

✓ chicken or turkey

✓ fish and mussels (these must be fresh, cooked, hot and eaten immediately).

The second type of iron is from **plant-sourced foods** and is called 'non-haem iron'. Good sources of this type of iron include:

✓ wholegrain breads and cereals (especially breakfast cereals with iron added)

✓ brewer's yeast (sprinkled over food)

✓ brown rice

✓ vegetables (peas) and legumes (dried beans), leafy green vegetables, broccoli

✓ dried fruit, nuts (almonds, cashews) and seeds (pumpkin and sesame seeds).

As iron found in plant-sourced foods is not as easily absorbed as the iron found in animal foods, you need to include a food which is high in vitamin C at the same meal to assist the iron absorption. For example, include one of the following at meal times: fruit juice, potatoes, tomatoes, fresh or dried fruit.

Pregnant women who are vegetarian need to take special care with their diet to ensure they have adequate iron intake and more importantly absorption. Even if you have not previously been a meat-eater, you may find when you are pregnant this changes and you start to crave red meat. This is a good example of the body's natural tendency to seek out that which it needs. If this is not an option, seek advice from your LMC or ask them to refer you to reputable information sources.

Zinc

Its role

Zinc is necessary for the functioning of more than 300 different enzymes, which means it plays a crucial role in a great number of bodily activities. The risk for zinc deficiency is greatest amongst pregnant and breastfeeding women, and so ensuring you have the correct level of zinc is important for all three phases of pre-conception, pregnancy and early childhood.

Although folic acid usually gets much attention because it helps prevent birth defects, zinc plays a key role in pregnancy as well, particularly in the final trimester, contributing to embryo and fetal development as well as to infant growth. The recommended dietary intake for non-pregnant women is 8mg, but during pregnancy and lactation this increases to 10–12 milligrams. Vegetarian women require more.

Effects of having too little

Low levels of zinc can reduce the amount of protein available to carry iron and vitamin A to the tissues, and it reduces mother's appetite and taste for foods. As a result, the growing fetus is at risk of inadequate growth and development, plus it often results in low birth-weight babies with a lowered immunity to infectious diseases.

General signs of a zinc deficiency are an under-performing immune system, increased susceptibility to infections, allergies, night blindness, loss of smell, hair loss, white spots under finger nails, skin problems, and sleep disturbances. Men with zinc shortage may have a problem with fertility, while women may experience irregular periods. Children with too little zinc may have stunted growth and slow sexual maturity.

Effects of having too much

Too much zinc interferes with metabolism and absorption of other important minerals in your body, specifically iron, magnesium and copper. An excessive amount of zinc can reduce immune function and reduce HDL (good cholesterol) levels.

Food sources

Zinc can be found in red meat, fish, pork, poultry, dairy products and fortified cereals. (Generally, zinc is found in the same foods in which you find iron, and similarly its absorption is better from animal-sourced foods than from plant-sourced foods.) Oysters are a good source, although as they fall into the shellfish category they should be avoided unless you can be sure they are fresh and cooked and served piping hot. Your LMC may recommend a pregnancy vitamin supplement that contains both the correct amounts of folic acid and zinc.

Iodine

Its role

Iodine is important for normal brain development, particularly for unborn babies, infants and young children. Pregnant and breastfeeding women need more iodine than the general population as they provide all of their baby's iodine. Pregnant women need a daily intake of 220 micrograms of the mineral, which is used by the thyroid to create a hormone which controls metabolism and digestion and also helps in the brain development of the fetus. Breastfeeding women require slightly more, at 270 micrograms per day.

Effects of having too little

Iodine deficiency is the single most common cause of preventable mental retardation and brain damage in the world. Too little dietary iodine can cause goitre or under-activity of the thyroid gland. Mild to moderate iodine deficiency can cause learning difficulties and affect physical development and hearing.

Effects of having too much

Large doses can be toxic, and in rare cases supplements can cause allergic reactions.

Food sources

Iodine is found in iodised table salt, bread, seafood, and dairy foods such as low-fat milk.

> # Important note for Australia and New Zealand
>
> In March 2008, Food Standards Australia New Zealand (FSANZ) introduced a food standard that required the replacement of non-iodised salt with iodised salt in most commercial bread production. This came into effect in October 2009. This action was taken to address the re-emergence of an iodine deficiency in Australia and New Zealand over the preceding decade. Those bakery products that fall outside the mandatory inclusion of iodised salt include: pizza bases, breadcrumbs, pastries, cakes, biscuits, organic and unleavened bread.

Magnesium

Its role

Magnesium is crucial for the body's utilisation of proteins, fats and carbohydrates, and helps build body tissue, including strong bones and teeth. It also regulates insulin and blood sugar levels, plus helps certain enzymes function properly. Research indicates that it may also control cholesterol and irregular heartbeats. Magnesium and calcium work in combination: magnesium relaxes muscles, while calcium stimulates muscles to contract.

When you are pregnant, magnesium helps build and repair your body tissue. A severe deficiency during pregnancy may lead to pre-eclampsia, birth defects, and infant mortality. Research suggests that proper levels of magnesium during pregnancy can help keep the uterus from contracting until week 35; dropping levels at this point may start labour contractions. Pregnant women need an intake of 350–360 milligrams of magnesium daily.

Effects of having too little

Magnesium deficiency is rare, but can cause weakness and, in extreme cases, convulsions.

Effects of having too much

This occurs usually as the result of taking an antacid or laxative high in magnesium. Large amounts may cause heart damage or respiratory failure; mild excess does not usually require treatment.

Food sources

Magnesium is found in many foods, including whole grains, nuts, meats, starches, milk, wheat bran, wheat germ, prawns, chickpeas, brazil nuts, almonds, wholemeal bread, chicken, seafood, pumpkin and sunflower seeds, and green leafy vegetables. A healthy varied diet should give you all the magnesium you need, although it is often contained in some prenatal vitamin supplements.

Pregnancy niggles

Constipation

During pregnancy constipation can occur from the effect of the hormone 'relaxin', pressure on your intestines from the baby growing, from high progesterone levels, or from taking iron supplements. If you are getting constipated, aid your body's uptake by splitting up your total iron supplement and taking it in several lots over the day, in between meals and with something containing vitamin C, like juice or fruit. Other methods of relieving constipation include eating foods rich in dietary fibre (whole grains, fruits and vegetables, and high-fibre breakfast cereal), and make sure you are exercising regularly and getting enough water to keep hydrated.

Nausea and morning sickness

Unfortunately these unpleasant symptoms are very common during the first trimester when hormones are coursing around your body. Another suggested reason is that the liver is working overnight to eliminate toxins which are present in your system on waking. As many a pregnant mum will attest, the waves of nausea are certainly not restricted to just the morning hours—it can and does strike at any time of the day.

Remedies differ depending on the person, but here are some to try.

❋ Eat something little, even if it is a cracker, toast, or a plain or ginger biscuit. If you hold off from eating, your blood sugar will drop even lower and you will probably find your nausea gets worse.

❋ Take small sips of iced water, flat lemonade or ginger ale.

❋ Talk to your LMC about B_6 supplements—these may alleviate nausea as it aids liver metabolism.

❋ Drink raspberry leaf, peppermint, and ginger root teas, as they have proven effective for some.

❋ Reduce fatty foods in your diet and increase carbohydrates, as this may be helpful.

❋ If you are taking a special pregnancy multivitamin and mineral formula and find you feel nauseous, try taking it later in the day with a meal.

Nausea may get in the way of your intention to exercise. If so, try eating a small snack before you attempt any activity. Exercise to the point of comfort and keep hydrated. If you are consistently nauseous at certain times of the day, try to slot in your exercise at times when you are not. Some women say that exercise actually helps them dissipate or avoid morning sickness altogether, but everyone is different, so listen to your body and adjust accordingly. The good news is that in most cases it tapers off by the end of the first trimester.

Heartburn and indigestion

Heartburn gives you a burning feeling in your oesophagus. This often occurs later in pregnancy and may be due to pregnancy hormones causing the relaxation of the sphincter muscle that closes off the stomach from the digestive tract increasing the reflux action. It is helpful to have smaller, more frequent meals, and to steer clear of foods that may be irritating, like spicy or greasy foods. Remain upright after eating, and try to not to have your evening meal too close to bedtime—allow a break of at least two to three hours before lights-out. Papaya enzymes can help alleviate pain and irritation from heartburn, so try papaya fruit or juice. Other remedies that may give relief are a glass of milk or a teaspoon of honey. You can also discuss possible pharmaceutical remedies with your LMC.

Cravings and aversions

Some pregnant women crave pickles and olives. One theory is that this could be due to a need for sodium, and during pregnancy adding a little salt to food is okay. Just go lightly with the salt shaker and don't be an 'aerial crop-duster'. Highly salted foods like chips and pretzels are best avoided or eaten occasionally as a treat food.

Some women develop a voracious sweet tooth, or crave dairy products.

Common aversions include alcohol, caffeinated drinks, meat, fatty foods, eggs and some strongly flavoured foods.

Key points

✗ **DON'TS**—raw eggs, shellfish, rare or raw meats, raw fish, pâté, deli cold meats and salads, smoking, alcohol, excess caffeine, non-prescription drugs and prescription drugs unless okayed by your LMC.

✓ **DO'S**—practise balance, variety and moderation with your healthy food intake. Reduce fats and sugars. Get enough folic acid via supplementation. Eat good nutritious wholesome food and stay well hydrated.

Chapter 3

The Fabulous, But So Often Forgotten, Pelvic Floor Muscles

Women and men both possess pelvic floor muscles, and both sexes need to ensure they stay in good working order. For women, however, this is of particular importance as 70% of those affected by incontinence are women. Pregnancy, childbirth, menopause and the anatomical structure of the female urinary tract account for this high incidence. By the end of reading this chapter I hope you will have completed at least one set of pelvic floor exercises, and that you will be a convert, wanting to make them an exercise habit for life.

Pelvic floor muscles

Put simply, the pelvic floor forms a sling of muscle that essentially keeps your pelvic organs in place and stops them falling out. They also kick in and provide a base of support whenever there is a sudden increase in intra-abdominal pressure; for example, when you cough. (Cough and see if you can feel that involuntary bounce of muscular support between your legs.)

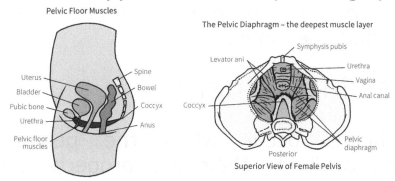

Fig.3.1

As pregnancy progresses, the pelvic floor muscles come under increasing strain, thanks to hormonal changes, weight gain and pressure downwards from the growing baby and uterus. They must provide support for nine months' gestation, then stretch to allow the passage of the baby through, and then bounce back into shape and return to normal function. A big ask indeed! So the more you can train and tone your pelvic floor muscles, the better able they will serve you on this journey and for life in general. Women over 35 should pay particular attention. The saying 'use it or lose it' certainly applies to an ageing pelvic floor region!

The pelvic floor muscles are attached in four main places: in the front to the pubic bone, at the rear to the tailbone at the base of the spine, and either side to the 'sit bones' or ischial tuberosities. If you cup your hands one on top of the other, this will give you a fair idea of the shape and size of the pelvic floor region. There are three outlets through the pelvic floor sling of muscle: the urethra, the vagina and the anus.

Stress incontinence

Problems occur when the pelvic floor muscles can't do their job properly because they are weak, stretched or torn, leading to possible urinary or even faecal leakage. The most typical problem women have to deal with is called 'stress incontinence'. That is the term used to describe involuntary urine leakage that can occur when someone with a weak pelvic floor region coughs, sneezes or exercises. It is most often preventable, but sadly remains a much more common problem than most people realise, largely due to women simply not being aware of the existence, function and regular exercising required of the pelvic floor.

The pelvic floor muscles are not the only means of support and continence control for this region; also playing an important part are the urethra, ligaments, and endopelvic fascia. In some cases, even with perfectly functioning pelvic floor muscles, women can still experience leakage. If this applies to you, then it is likely that the incontinence is linked to some dysfunction of these other structures, in which case seeking expert investigation, advice and treatment is recommended. (See helpful websites and contacts at the conclusion of this chapter.)

Here is a way to understand the how the pelvic floor muscles and other structures work together. Imagine a boat tied up at a wharf: the boat represents your uterus, bladder and bowel, the ropes to tether it to the wharf are the supporting ligaments, and the sea level corresponds to how strong and effective your pelvic floor muscles are. A strong, toned pelvic floor keeps the boat level, nestled into the wharf with ropes taut; however, if the water level is low (a saggy weak pelvic floor), then the drag and strain goes on the tether ropes and everything attached.

Incidence

Some type of stress incontinence is experienced by 20–30% of women—that's around ONE in four!

The following factors increase the chances of incontinence:

✳ **Having given birth** The number of vaginal deliveries experienced by a woman increases the risk of incontinence among women in younger (under 65 years) age groups.

✳ **Age** Although the prevalence of incontinence rises with age, there is no clear evidence that age *in itself* leads to a higher risk of incontinence—it is not an inevitable aspect of ageing.

   ✳ **Obesity** This is an independent risk factor for incontinence.

   ✳ **Constipation** This may be a risk factor for urinary incontinence.

Pelvic floor exercises

Rationale for strengthening pelvic floor muscles

The pelvic floor muscles which lie at the outlet of the pelvis are intimately involved with the birth process, especially during the second stage of labour. These muscles must be able to stretch and recoil with each contraction of the uterus, and in doing so aid the baby's passage down and through the birth canal. This natural process stretches them to a weakened state, and after birth they don't just ping back, so they need attention—and fast.

There is no doubt that performing pelvic floor exercises before, during and after pregnancy is beneficial. It is the one workout where you can be exercising away and not get up a sweat! In fact you can be performing a pelvic floor workout on the bus, while having a conversation with someone, even while waiting in the supermarket checkout queue. Brilliant!

No exercise attire or equipment required! An added bonus to toned pelvic floor muscles is that they can enhance your sex life. Poor vaginal tone can create a lack of sensation for you and your partner, but by exercising these muscles regularly you can avoid that. Once you have mastered the exercise you can even test out your 'squeeze strength' during sex.

Kegels

Dr Arnold Kegel was one of the first to describe how to do pelvic floor muscle exercises in the 1940s, hence his name being used to describe the process. This means you will probably find the term 'kegel' used in American publications—'do a kegel', 'kegel muscles', even 'kegeling'—whereas in New Zealand and Australia we usually refer to them as the pelvic floor.

How to do them

For many women, step one is finding out where their pelvic floor muscles actually are and what it feels like to do a contraction of those muscles.

The exercise

You can do pelvic floor exercises in any position, but let us start with sitting, and as the muscles get stronger you can progress to standing.

1. Squeeze or tighten and draw in and up around your anus (back passage), vagina and urethra (bladder outlet).

2. LIFT UP inside and try to HOLD this contraction STRONGLY for as long as you can (3–5 seconds). KEEP BREATHING!

3. Now release and RELAX. You should have a definite feeling of letting go. Congratulations—you have just done a pelvic floor contraction.

4. Rest 5–10 seconds, then repeat steps 1–3 again, always putting a rest in between each contraction.

You will feel your lower abdominal muscles tightening a little, too, as they work in partnership with the pelvic floor, but focus on lifting the pelvic floor up first; the lower abdominals are just a willing accomplice.

Good form

Good form is not holding your breath, not pushing down, but pulling your abdominals in tightly while tightening your buttocks and thighs. A few good contractions are more beneficial than many half-hearted ones. Remember to use the muscles when you need them most: before you cough, sneeze, lift, bend, jump or get up out of a chair.

The PF 'mantra'
   LIFT, SQUEEZE, HOLD, RELAX.
   8–12 CONTRACTIONS, 3 TIMES A DAY

Visualisations
   It does not matter if initially you can only manage a squeeze of a second or two, as with regular workouts you will quickly build up endurance and tone. Visualisation can really help.

Visualisation 1
   Imagine your pelvic floor muscles act like a lift in a building. Close the door, rise up a few floors. Let the doors open again. Don't hold your breath. Now do 5–10 more.

Visualisation 2 (more advanced)
   Close those lift doors, rise up to the 5th floor, let the passengers file out slowly, then slowly let the lift return to the ground floor. Do it again and remember to breathe evenly throughout the manoeuvre. Repeat 5–10 times. If you find it easy to hold, try to hold longer and repeat as many as you are able. Work towards 12 long, strong holds.

Trouble?
   If you are having trouble finding or feeling the muscles, try stopping your urine mid-flow. This will allow you to experience a pelvic floor

contraction. This is fine to do as an initial way of isolating the muscles and getting a sense of their action, but please don't get into the habit of stopping mid-stream regularly. You should always encourage full emptying of the bladder to avoid any chance of bladder infections. Conversely, when the bladder and bowel empty there is a definite relaxing of the pelvic floor muscles. If you are unable to feel a definite squeeze or lift, you may have very weak pelvic floor muscles, and in almost all cases it is possible to retrain them. If you continue to have concerns, you can always contact a professional for advice. Refer to your local helpline number and website at the end of this chapter.

When to do them

Before giving birth

On the whole this is one muscle that does not need a rest day. If you achieve a few minutes of exercising the pelvic floor each and every day you will be doing exactly what is needed to maintain good tone. It is a misconception that a strong pelvic floor could hinder the birth of your baby—provided you know how to *relax* the muscles as well. Research also shows that women who regularly exercise their pelvic floor muscles often have a shorter second stage (that is, the pushing the baby out part of labour). The best advice is that any strengthening and tightening of these muscles should always involve a corresponding relaxation phase. A strong, toned set of pelvic floor muscles are more flexible than flaccid weak ones, and that's the key: flexibility.

I met a lady who was fastidious about doing pelvic floor exercises, and she practised them daily throughout her entire pregnancy. She was also very fit and active. However, she had no concept of relaxing those little muscles, so when it came to pushing her baby out she encountered trouble as she couldn't 'turn off' the tightening and lifting up feeling.

In the third trimester

You may find in the final few weeks of pregnancy that you experience a bit of stress incontinence. This is normal due to the sheer weight and pressure of the baby pushing down on that region, plus the effect on the muscles and ligaments of a pregnancy hormone flooding around your body called relaxin. So if you do get a little leakage, rest assured it need only be a temporary thing and use it to galvanise you even more into getting those pelvic floor muscles working.

After giving birth

This will be the first exercise you will do after giving birth. In all seriousness, you can attempt pelvic floor exercises the very next day.

You may wish to do your first set sitting on the toilet, and you may only feel a flicker of activity, if anything. Rest assured, they will bounce back if you keep at it. The body has remarkable powers of recovery and, although it may feel as if nothing is happening, you are sending messages to the muscle fibres and they will respond.

Even if you have had a caesarean section it is still possible to experience a weak pelvic floor due to the weight of the baby pressing down in the final trimester.

If you have perineal damage, whether through a planned cut (episiotomy) or through tearing, these exercises will speed up the healing process, as they bring improved blood flow to the wound, so—JUST DO IT. Each time you do a set of pelvic floor exercises, do the most you can. It won't happen overnight, but improvement will happen. If you put in the effort, and with regular attention, you should see positive results in a matter of weeks.

Mind over matter

When your pelvic floor muscles are weak, as you will experience in the days immediately after giving birth, you may need to consciously think about squeezing them when you need them most; for example, when you go to cough, sneeze or get up out of a chair.

The muscle action will, with repetition, become automatic, but initially you may need to provide a mental kick-start to make sure they contract when you need them to.

Use it or lose it—for life

Studies done in the past five years conclude that 'providing pelvic floor muscle education and encouragement of exercises during pregnancy and after birth is effective in preventing incontinence six months later.' However, the research also says this effect may not last several years later. So if you don't continue doing your pelvic floor exercises regularly, don't expect to have a toned, taut and terrific pelvic floor. Doing a few flickering squeezes as you read this chapter and then forgetting about it will not bring about any positive or lasting change. This is a sling of muscle that needs to be worked out—daily—for life. It's quite simple: use it or lose it.

Find something you do regularly that you can link these exercises to, so you remember to do them each and every day, like turning on a tap, opening the fridge door, or waiting in your car at the traffic lights. Link doing a set of 10 with a smiley sticker, and plaster a few around the house in places that will catch your eye; for example, on a door handle, on the toothbrush container or inside the fridge door. I often do my pelvic floor exercises when I am stretching or when sitting at my desk working on the computer. It doesn't matter the time of day, what you are wearing or who you are with, just get squeezing. If all else fails, do a set when you tumble into bed at night before you drift off to sleep.

Spread the word

We all need to do pelvic floor exercises in order to maintain their strength and function for the rest of our lives. Not getting your pelvic floor muscles functioning effectively following childbirth could potentially spell bigger problems later on in life. Some older women (aged 50+) who suffer prolapses of organs like the bladder and vagina may have been able to prevent it happening had they adopted the habit of regular pelvic floor exercises following childbirth.

Now that you know the benefit and importance of this pelvic floor workout, why don't you have a chat to those women in your life who you think may need extra encouragement to get active in this domain. Maybe your mother or grandmother might have been of the generation when it was not talked about or not emphasised as critically important for their future physical health.

Ongoing continence problems

The pelvic floor muscles are important to a women's ability to stay dry, but they are not the only reason for incontinence occurring. Issues of incontinence can be frustrating and embarrassing, but crucially there is good help available. It is certainly not something that women have to suffer. So if you experience any form of incontinence or urgency to get to the toilet after childbirth, then seek professional advice.

Start by ringing the free-phone numbers of your country's Continence Association:

Australian Continence Association
1800-33-00-66
Website www.continence.org.au

New Zealand Continence Association
0800-650-659
Website www.continence.org.nz

You could also ask your doctor for a referral to a continence professional, who is usually a physiotherapist specialising in pelvic floor management.

A word of caution for élite athletes

New Zealand research by Jennifer Ann Kruger of the University of Auckland investigated observations that élite athletes seemed to have a prolonged hard time in second stage labour (the process of pushing the baby out) that often resulted in an intervention by the LMC, or even caesarean section. For the purpose of this research, 'élite athletes' were defined as those women who had been exercising to an extremely high level daily for over five years, in activities that involved regular, repeated landing or impact (for example, top-level netballers, runners, triathletes, dancers, gymnasts, etc).

Kruger found that while it is not possible to say unequivocally that élite athletes have a hard time in labour—based on this latest information, which was gathered from a small sample of women and combined with interviews with their pregnancy caregivers—the evidence so far suggests that they may. The study examined the actual pelvic floor muscles involved in the birth process, which showed changes in both form and function. Intense high-impact exercise involves repetitive pelvic floor muscle floor contraction—far more than the normal population would do—and the muscles in these women studied had adapted to become very tight and strong.

The advice from this research to super-fit pregnant athletes, to enable better pregnancy outcomes, is to cut back on the high-impact exercise, and crucially try to learn how to *relax and release* the pelvic floor muscles, or at least learn to feel the difference between a contraction and no contraction. For élite athletes it would seem the ability to relax the pelvic floor proves difficult, but if mastered this could help with their second stage labour. Also, this group of women must discuss with their LMC that they have been or are continuing to participate in exercise at an élite level.

(Based on Jennifer Ann Kruger, 'Pelvic Floor Muscle Function in Élite Nulliparous Athletes', a thesis submitted in fulfilment of the requirements for the degree of Doctor of Philosophy, Department of Sport and Exercise Science, University of Auckland, 2008.)

Key points

○ Do some pelvic floor exercises. Make it a regular occurrence, but don't do to excess.

○ Make sure you can tighten the muscle, but also consciously release the muscle (useful in the 'bearing down' phase of delivery).

○ If you are a regular exerciser, you will have some pelvic floor tone established already, so just do a maintenance level.

○ If you haven't exercised before, get your pelvic floor muscles active, but remember the balance between tightening and releasing.

○ Start pelvic floor exercises from day one, after birth. You may only feel a flicker of response, but it's the start you need. Increase in intensity and number over the next few weeks to re-establish tone and flexibility.

Chapter 4

Your Crucial Core

Core muscles

The core is the bony framework and musculature that makes up your trunk. It is the region between your left and right shoulder, and left and right hip, encompassing both the front and back of your body, with your spine acting as a central reinforcing rod. The muscles that are commonly referred to as 'core muscles' are the abdominals and back muscles; and to a lesser extent, but still involved in core movements, are the chest and buttock muscles.

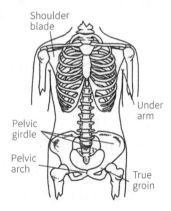

Fig 4.1 Key core bony structure

You could compare the role of the body's core to the core of an apple—it is the central supporting structure to which the rest of the bits attach, in the body's case the arms, legs, neck and head. A strong core equals a sturdy, resilient body. A weak core sets you up for an increased chance of aches and pain and possibly even injury when you ask 'more' of your body. Core strengthening is especially important before, during and after pregnancy, as it is specifically this region of your body that undergoes huge physical change, expanding over the pregnancy to accommodate your growing baby.

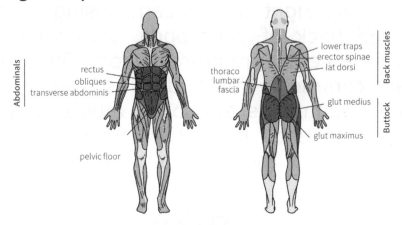

Fig 4.2 Key core muscles

The term 'core' has only really become commonly used in mainstream exercising in the past decade; increasingly so in recent years with a greater focus on prevention of injury and functional fitness. Nonetheless, you have been using your core whether you were aware of it or not, as these are the muscles that come into play in everyday activities. For example, just walking on uneven ground gets the core muscles working to stabilise you and stop you from falling over; balancing while standing on one foot fires up the core muscles; even more mundane chores like hanging out the washing, bringing in the shopping bags, and bending down to pick up children all involve some degree of core muscle activity. These muscles are the body's unsung heroes.

You will be using those muscles like never before as a new-time mum, and this could spell a recipe for disaster. Take one set of weak abdominals, mix in weak back muscles, then combine with repetitive lifting and twisting (as you will be doing with a new baby), and—hey presto—you have likely got yourself some back pain! So in this chapter we will look at how you can safely strengthen your core muscles, and adopt safe lifting techniques. In each of the trimester chapters, the sample workout will contain appropriate core strengthening exercises.

Rationale for strengthening core muscles

As women age they can tend to become less flexible and the core muscles weaken. The core forms your powerhouse for smooth functional movement, so in your thirties and forties, pregnant or not, this is the sort of exercising that really pays dividends. However, during pregnancy it is even more important because you are dealing with an ever-changing weight distribution, resulting in your centre of gravity moving; because of this, you need both awareness and stability of the body's core to minimise or prevent back pain and injury. It is estimated that 9 out of 10 women experience some level of back pain during pregnancy, ranging from an annoying niggle to continual debilitating discomfort. Core strengthening is one of the best things you can do to minimise your chance of suffering such pain, by providing good muscular support for your spine. Addressing and improving the elements of balance and strength of your core musculature gives you not only quality of movement, but also quality of life.

Some of you will already have other young children and will no doubt be familiar with the incessant 'up up up' that a toddler calls out to mum. Being a mum involves an extraordinary amount of lifting, bending, twisting and carrying. On any given day you could be repetitively lifting the baby, the capsule, the pram and any or all of the paraphernalia that goes with moving from point A to point B with a little one. The best way to protect your back and allow you to be the active mum you want to be is to have strong core muscles that switch on and do their job when required.

It is worth focusing on all the lifting and carrying that a new mum does, because it wasn't until I was a first-time mum that I fully understood how physically demanding that first 6–12 months really is. With my firstborn son, Ben, I was in reasonably fit shape post-birth, but I suffered from back pain caused by a lapse when lifting and incorrectly using my back 'as a crane'. If I can help you strengthen your back now, before giving birth and possibly prevent you from getting back strain, then it is worth banging on about it, I hope you agree.

Let us consider what you are actually demanding of your body when lifting a baby through to a toddler who weighs approximately 10 kilograms. You bend over, you pick up the baby (or possibly a struggling toddler), which may involve you twisting and lifting, and then most likely you balance that weight asymmetrically on your hip. It happens so frequently during the day that you won't even give it a thought—that is, until you've got a sore back and it becomes painful to do so.

Time-efficient training

Core strengthening exercises can be very time-efficient, because you are strengthening a bunch of muscles in one exercise rather than isolating and training each individual muscle as you would with more traditional gym weight machine exercises. Unlike bicep curls or leg extensions, you typically don't *see* a lot of external muscle contraction when you train the core, as the stabilising muscles are located deep in the body around the bones and joints of the spine, shoulder girdle and pelvis.

Core strengthening isn't about developing muscle size, it is about improving functional muscle strength for everyday activities, making your body resilient for physical activity. And let's face it, in the time-strapped, baby-centric world you are about to enter, having a time-efficient form of strength training is a must, otherwise even with best intentions you just won't find the time to do it. Concentrate the time you *do* have on core strengthening exercises to minimise injury and maximise efficient movement. The exercises don't require expensive equipment and are easy to do at home, as you mainly use your own body weight against gravity with perhaps a Swiss ball to further stimulate balance and stabilisation.

Core is key

Aside from during pregnancy, core exercises are valuable for your general fitness. The push-button, drive-through, remote-controlled, less labour-intensive lifestyle that most of us lead has driven us away from naturally and habitually using our core muscles. Compared with our parents and their parents, we sit more and lead a largely automated life. Technology is great for so many reasons, but where it can be a negative influence in our lives is when it minimises how much we move. Our bodies are designed for movement and function best when we are fit and active on a daily basis. At any stage of your life, strengthening your core musculature should be a valuable part of your overall fitness, and specifically will improve the flexibility and function of your back, improve your posture and make you less susceptible to back aches and injury.

Core and posture

Core stability and posture are inextricably linked. A strong, stable core enhances good posture. During pregnancy, how you hold yourself will naturally adjust to accommodate your changing shape and weight as your uterus and baby grow. The relaxing and loosening effect of the pregnancy hormones on your ligament and joints also makes you more susceptible to sagging, poor posture. What was a small lower back curve can become exaggerated as your tummy extends forwards. This can put extra strain on your already stretched abdominals and more stress on your spine. Heavier, fuller breasts can cause you to round your shoulders and slump forwards, which in turn forces your chin to jut forward, placing extra stress down the back of your neck

114

(cervical spine). Due to your increasing weight, you will probably stand with your feet wider apart for balance, and that in itself can apply different stresses to the hips and lower back. Core strengthening exercises will help minimise and alleviate the postural strain and stresses on your pregnant body.

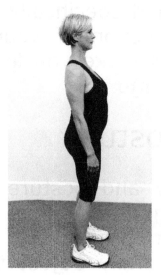

Fig.4.3 Good posture and alignment when pregnant

Your spine has four curves, three moveable, one fixed. Beginning at the top, the concave curve of the neck moving down to the slightly convex curve of the upper back, then to the concave curve of the lower back, and finally the fixed convex curve of the triangular bone that forms the rear wall of the pelvis—the sacrum. These curves are essential to the spine being able to function well. Good posture does not attempt to eliminate the curves; instead, it should eliminate any exaggeration, and aim for balance between them. Erect upright posture improves your health and wellbeing, your muscles function better, you are able to breathe deeper and your self-esteem will be boosted by a confident stance.

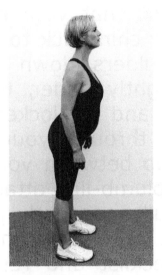

Fig.4.4 Poor postural position when pregnant

Be aware of how you stand, walk, sit and lift during pregnancy. A little care and self-correction in order to maintain good posture can really help you avoid discomfort. Not many of us have perfect posture to begin with, so if you have been out of alignment for years, then correcting yourself is going to initially feel weird. Correcting little and often is the key, so every time you pass a mirror do a quick 'self-check and restack'.

Standing smart when pregnant

Working down the body from your head to the feet, run through this postural alignment for good standing posture.

Chin tucked so that your eyes are looking forward, slid your chin back towards your spine (retraction), shoulders down and back, tuck your tailbone slightly under, feet hip distance apart, knees soft and not locked into extension. Finally, lengthen through your mid-section by extending the gap between your ribs and hips. Try imagining a plumb-line attached to the very apex of your skull and gently pulling you up a few centimetres. It is often not until you go through this checklist and restack your body that you realise how slumped you actually were. The next time you are standing in a queue at the supermarket or petrol station—*stop, check and restack.*

Sitting smart when pregnant

You may think that slouching on a couch is resting your body, but that is not the case when it comes to your lower back. Sloppy sitting puts a lot of pressure on the discs in your back; the spongy bits between the bony vertebrae. Lying applies the least amount of disc pressure; when standing the disc pressure is four times greater than in lying, but when sitting it is a whopping 16 times higher. That is why when you have a sore back, sitting is one of the worst positions to be in for any length of time, as any increased disc pressure can exacerbate discomfort.

However, sitting is something we do a lot every day and that's not going to change, so here's how to sit smart. Your anchor points are your sit bones (ischial tuberosities). Beware of sitting evenly on your sit bones, as the process of elongating and stacking your spine correctly starts right from the sit bones and continues all the way up to the top of your neck. Be aware of maintaining the small natural curve in your lower back. Try using a small pillow, lumbar roll or rolled-up towel to help you maintain that natural lower back curve, and make sure you shuffle your butt to the back of the seat. Then 'sit tall' by lifting your rib cage away from your pelvis, creating a sense of elongation in your mid-region. Finally, roll your shoulders back and down. Long car trips or plane flights can be particularly troublesome for backs, so if you are travelling for any length of time use a lower back arch support as suggested above.

Interesting opposites

Correcting and maintaining good alignment in both sitting and standing require opposite pelvic movements.

* **standing**—correct the typical forward tilt by tucking your buttocks under slightly

* **sitting**—correct the typical backward tilt by arching your lower back slightly.

Lifting smart when pregnant

You have already read about the focus on good lifting for new mums. Here is the low-down on how to lift safely. Think first: plan your lift. Squat down, pull the load close to your body and keep it there. Bend your knees, and power upward using your large leg muscles to take the load. Never twist and lift. If you want to change direction, move your feet, not your back. The 'straw that broke the camel's back' is often lifting the baby in a capsule/baby seat in and out of the car. So be aware that the specific lifting required by a new mum puts you at risk of damaging your back, mainly because the baby capsule move involves both load and rotation.

It only takes a second or two to pause first and to get yourself in the best possible position. Get as close as possible to what you are about to lift, draw in and brace your lower abdominals to provide support to your lower back, and whenever possible bend, and use your large leg muscles to take the weight of the load, keeping your back as upright as you can. You could rest your knee on the rear seat when you are leaning into the car to ease the load. The more you do this routine of pause, check, brace then lift, the more automatic it will become and the safer your lifting will be.

Abdominals—a vital part of core support

As you have seen on the diagram identifying the core muscles, the abdominals are a vital part of our core trunk support, and that certainly applies during pregnancy.

On the face of it, abdominal exercises during pregnancy might seem a waste of time when that is where your body is going to expand enormously as the baby grows—and you don't want the muscles to squash and hurt the growing baby.

The role of abdominals in pregnancy

Nonetheless, it *is* advisable to do some form of abdominal exercises throughout all three trimesters, even though of course this will modify as your pregnancy progresses. Abdominal tone will give some support for the increasing weight of your uterus and give necessary postural support for your spine, helping prevent and minimise back pain. Toned abdominals will also help you push your baby out during the second stage of labour, and allow you to get your pre-pregnancy shape back more quickly following the birth. You won't be strengthening the particular set of abdominal muscles that run down the centre of your stomach, though; rather you will focus on the deep abdominals and those on either side of your body called the obliques (see the detailed description below). From about the second trimester on—when your baby bump is clearly expanding forwards—you will no longer do any curling forward or sit-up style abdominal exercising and you should be aware of a 'diastasis' appearing (tummy muscle gap) (Fig.4.7).

Modified appropriate abdominal exercises as shown in this book will not 'squash' or harm your growing baby. During pregnancy your abdominals provide a muscular corset around your vital organs and your growing baby. Having toned, strong abdominals throughout all three trimesters contributes to a strong central core that, while stretching to accommodate the baby's change in size and weight, provides necessary stability and support.

But first let's look at what makes up the abdominal muscle group.

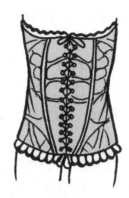

Fig.4.5

The abdominals

The abdominals are a set of muscles that work together to allow you to twist, turn and bend forwards. Let us start with the deepest level of muscle which is often rated as the most important one!

✳ **Transverse abdominis** Often called the **corset muscle** and for good reason, as it sits the deepest out of the four layers of abdominal muscles that hold in and support your organs. It is the only layer of the abdominal muscles that attaches via fascia to each level of the lumbar spine. Strengthening this horizontal layer of muscle will provide support for the spine as well as for the pelvic floor. A weak transverse abdominis sets you up for back pain in pregnancy. If your abdominal foundation isn't strong, then as your baby grows bigger and heavier there will be a lot of extra pull and stress on ligaments and joints leading to aches and pains.

✳ **Internal obliques** Running from the pelvis on an angle up to the lower ribs and into the centre of the body, these muscles on either side of the spine are the next layer up from the transverse abdominis, but still contribute to core stability. They work in partnership with their sister muscle group, the external obliques, and their action is to create twisting (rotation) and bending (sideways).

✳ **External obliques** Running from the lateral ribs down towards the centre of your abdomen, these muscles are again involved in twisting (rotation) and bending (sideways). The internal and external obliques help define your waist—remember this for when you are no longer pregnant, as you will be waving goodbye to any discernible waist from about your second trimester on!

✳ **Rectus abdominis** This top layer of muscle runs from the breast bone to the pubic bone. It consists of two muscles running vertically and joined in the middle by a thin strip of connective tissue—the 'linea alba'. The rectus is the muscle that is activated primarily when doing sit-ups or 'crunches'. Overworking this superficial muscle while ignoring the deeper layers and obliques can actually give you a strong but bulbous-looking abdomen. You may have heard people referring to exercising their upper or lower abdominals. This terminology is misleading as the rectus is one continuous sheet of muscle and you can't exercise the upper or lower portions separately. You can do exercises that emphasise the upper part or the lower part of the muscle, but the whole muscle will still contract. Remember from the second trimester on, you will not be doing *any* curling up abdominal exercises that target the rectus muscle.

You may also hear the term **'deep abdominals':** this refers to the transverse abdominis in conjunction with the internal obliques; the two deepest layers. These are the vital abdominals to keep toned throughout pregnancy for the major prevention of back pain.

Expansion of waistline

You can expect to gain many extra centimetres around your middle as your baby grows, with an average weight gain of about 10–12 kilograms. Not only will the abdominal muscles stretch to accommodate this growth, but the band of tissue running up the midline of your stomach muscles from pubic bone to the bottom of the breast bone—the linea alba—will also stretch apart to give your baby more room. That wonderful hormone relaxin also plays its part in softening the linea alba.

How much the linea alba separates differs in each woman, but it can be anywhere up to 4 centimetres and it all begins at the end of your first trimester at around 12 weeks. This gap between your superficial abdominals is called the 'diastasis'. The process is certainly not painful, it happens slowly and it occurs with most women, to varying degrees, although a regular regime of abdominal exercises may lessen the amount it separates.

Due to this expanded connective tissue (remember it is not muscle), it is important not to strain this area when it is in this temporary but relatively stretched and weakened state. Forward sit-ups and rotational abdominal exercises should be avoided from the second trimester onwards, as the movements can contribute to an increased diastasis. Since you will have less abdominal strength for movements like getting up out of a chair or getting out of bed, you will need to adapt slightly by doing a small roll to the side and then using your leg muscles to get you into standing position.

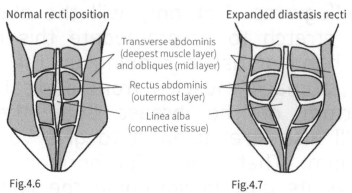

Normal recti position

Expanded diastasis recti

Transverse abdominis (deepest muscle layer) and obliques (mid layer)

Rectus abdominis (outermost layer)

Linea alba (connective tissue)

Fig.4.6   Fig.4.7

The presence of the diastasis (tummy muscle gap) means the balance of core stability is now changed, resulting in less support for your pelvis and back and more work for your back muscles. The gap can run above and/or below the belly button, and may be slightly different in each woman. Knowing how to test for a diastasis is important following the birth. It is not particularly important beforehand, but just be aware that you probably will have a gap, especially if this is a second or subsequent pregnancy.

Core stability exercises

These are basic core strengthening exercises. In each trimester chapter I will also incorporate appropriate core strengthening exercises for that stage of pregnancy into the sample workout.

If you are past 16 weeks pregnant, you can briefly try the neutral spine exercise, but, as it's advisable not to be on your back for any extended length of time, you will need to skip to those which are positioned on hands and knees or standing.

What you need

Some cushioning for under your body when lying on the floor, like a towel for carpeted floors, or a rubber mat for a hard surface.

Neutral spine

Neutral spine is a stable, safe position for your pelvis and lower back, and is the starting position for most core-strengthening exercises. Once you know where 'neutral' is for you, you can adopt it in sitting or standing positions, but let us begin in a lying position.

Lying on your back, knees bent with feet flat on the floor. (If after 16 weeks' pregnancy, start with standing abdominal bracing or four-point kneeling, explained below.) Neutral spine is the position midway between a lower back arch or extension and lower back rounding or flexion. It stabilises the lower back region by having the vertebral discs in a safe, uncompressed position. Depending on your body shape, you may be able to slide your fingers into a very slight gap beneath your lower back when lying. How much gap? Imagine just a whisper of air can get through, or there is space for just one grape to sit in between your lower back and the floor without being squashed. To find this midway point, flatten your back into the floor so you can feel the mat, then do an exaggerated arch off the mat. Do a few pelvic movements or tilts as described, then allow your pelvis to settle back to neutral – midway in between, neither tipped up nor dropped down.

Neutral spine, adding 'abdominal bracing'

Abdominal tightening or 'bracing' is the activation of the deep transverse abdominis muscles. The bracing action is when you draw your tummy muscles in towards your spine, aiming for tension across the area like a taunt trampoline. It is *not* a push-out action resulting in your abdominals being more like a bouncy castle. Once you have mastered the 'draw in and brace' action, you will find it invaluable throughout your pregnancy (even with an expanding belly), as it provides support for your spine as well as your growing baby. With neutral spine, exhale and lift up your pelvic floor muscles (always get into the habit of lifting up your pelvic floor muscles at the same time), then draw your bellybutton towards your spine and imagine your two hip bones drawing together at the same time. Think of it like a three-way zip action: zip up your pelvic floor, and then zip in your abdominals from either side so that you now have firm support across your lower abdomen. Avoid holding your breath.

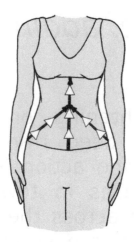

Fig.4.8 Zip it up

Your deep abdominals are now activated, and you should be able to feel this tension in the muscle by pressing your fingers just inside your hip bones. If you are having problems identifying the muscle, release and relax and then cough, and you should feel the muscle slightly bounce out under your fingertips. This is purely to allow you to locate the muscle, as the action of bracing as emphasised above is all about drawing *inwards* and creating a firm tension. Hold it for a count of 5–10, then gently release (unzip) both the pelvic floor and the abdominals. Important form points are to initiate the contraction on an exhaling breath, as this eliminates unnecessary tension and activation of the chest and diaphragm. Continue to breathe evenly throughout while maintaining the contraction. Make sure you are not flattening your back into the floor. The muscle contraction is strong, but there is very little movement of the spine.

Neutral spine, abdominal bracing, adding leg movements

Progress the above exercise by adding leg movements while maintaining the position and deep abdominal contraction. Establish neutral spine, draw in and brace your abdominals, exhale and slide one foot out along the floor, extend your leg only as far as you can maintain the neutral spine position, then inhale and draw the foot in again. You can place your fingertips on your hip bones to make sure there is no movement or titling of your pelvis. Alternate legs and repeat 10–15 times slowly and smoothly on each side.

Progress again by bringing one leg up at a time into a lifted table-top position, then slowly lower one leg at a time. Up, up, down, down. Remember to maintain your pelvis position; your tummy must not bulge out. Repeat 10–15 times on each side. The correct breathing to go with this exercise would be: exhale and lift the leg, inhale, exhale to lift the other leg, inhale, exhale to lower the leg, inhale, exhale to lower the other leg.

Standing abdominal bracing

You can do the same abdominal bracing in a standing position, too. Stand feet hip-distance apart with an upright posture. As you breathe out, do the three-way zip manoeuvre by drawing your belly button towards your spine, and drawing those two hip bones together. Your lower back may flatten just slightly, but the focus of the movement is the deep abdominals contracting, not the spine rounding. Hold it for 5–10 seconds and then release. Some women find it helps to envision this movement as 'hugging their baby' in towards the spine. This abdominal 'draw in and brace' is part of a good preparation for lifting.

Four-point kneeling—stabilisation of pelvis and shoulder girdles, adding abdominal bracing (Fig.4.9)

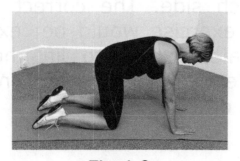

Fig.4.9

On hands and knees, in a square table-top position, weight equally distributed, elbows soft and lengthen through the back of the neck. Let your belly relax without moving the spine or the pelvis, then, as you exhale, zip up your pelvic floor and gently pull your belly button up towards your spine. There should be no movement in your spine or pelvis, and the buttocks are not involved. Keep breathing evenly and hold the contraction for 5–10 seconds, then release.

Three-point kneeling, adding one limb lift (Figs 4.10, 4.11)

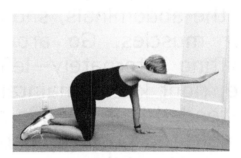

Fig.4.10

Progress the above exercise by lifting one point of your stable base off the floor, keeping your weight evenly distributed between your three supporting limbs.

Begin by lifting one hand off the floor and extend the arm out in front of you, making sure you maintain your body position without any movement in any direction.

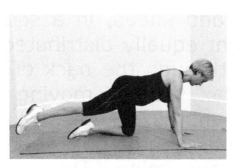

Fig.4.11

Now try lifting one knee, extend your leg out behind you. As your weight shifts, your body will try to move to the side, especially when you lift a lower limb, but try hard to minimise this shift as much as possible by engaging those stabilising core muscles around your hips and shoulders. This exercise is strengthening the abdominals, shoulder, hip and back extensor muscles. Go around the four 'table legs', lifting alternately—left arm, right arm, left knee, right knee—maintaining a static hold of the extended limb for five seconds then returning to table top position in between. The higher towards horizontal you extend your arm or leg, the harder the exercise becomes. The less body movement the better.

Two-point kneeling, adding two limb lifts (Fig.4.12)

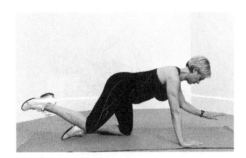

Fig.4.12

Progress the above exercise further, by extending diagonal limbs. With abdominals drawn in and braced, extend the opposite arm and knee on the diagonal while holding stable your trunk's table-top position. Extend your right arm forwards and left leg back, hold for five seconds, then return back to table-top. Then do the other diagonal. Keep breathing evenly. Repeat 10–15 times each side.

Side-lying, adding hip lift (Fig.4.13)

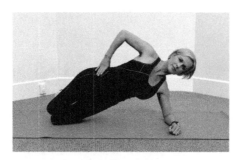

Fig.4.13

Lie on your side, legs bent behind your body, your thighs and torso in line, upper body weight off the floor, supported on your bent elbow which is sitting under your shoulder. Lift your hips up, maintaining a straight body-line from your lower shoulder to your knees. Hold for 5–10 seconds, then lower. Do a set of 10, then roll over and do the same on the other side.

Plank, half- and full—static contraction of core muscles

Note: Full planks can be performed in the first trimester only, half-planks in the first and second trimesters. Do not perform the face-down plank exercise in trimester three, as the weight of your baby bump will put too much strain on the lower back area.

Half-plank (first and second trimesters) (Fig.4.14)

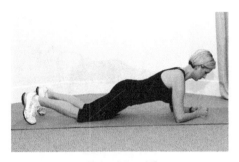

Fig.4.14

Lying face down, elbows tucked under your upper body and ribcage, keeping your back in neutral, zip up, draw in and brace your abdominals, then push up to support your body weight from your knees to your forearms. Tuck your tailbone under and squeeze your buttocks. Keep your lower legs on the ground, and maintain your body straight and firm 'like a plank', with no sagging in the middle, and with your spine in line from your neck to the base of your pelvis. Maintain the position for 10–20 seconds, keep breathing steadily throughout, then lower to the floor. Once you are able to complete a set of 10 half-planks, then you can progress to the full plank.

Full plank (first trimester only) (Fig.4.15)

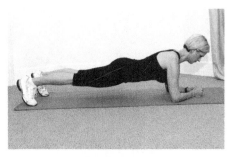

Fig.4.15

Lying on your stomach, tuck your toes under, draw in and brace your abdominals, and push up onto your feet. Tuck your tailbone under and squeeze your buttocks, keeping your spine in line and body firm like a rigid plank from head to toes. Again start with 10 seconds and build up to 20, and then a minute. Breathe evenly throughout.

Using a Swiss ball for exercising core muscles

A large inflatable ball (Swiss ball) is also effective in strengthening the core as, because it is round, it is a very unstable base that forces your core muscles to fire to help you maintain your balance and position. It gets its name due to its origins, but it is also known as a fit ball, a physio ball, a birth ball and a stability ball. The Swiss connection came about way back in the 1960s when a Swiss spinal rehabilitation specialist, Dr Susan Klein-Vogelbach, wanted a piece of equipment to help her orthopaedic patients re-educate their movement. She asked an Italian toy-maker to see if he could come up with something suitable that would support the weight of an adult, and so the Swiss ball was devised.

Using a Swiss ball encourages you to use your body as a whole in three-dimensional movements, which is far more functional than the single-plane movements typically experienced on traditional weight machines. As with any new skill, don't expect or attempt too much the first few times you use the ball—you will not be an expert immediately. In fact, most people probably feel quite unco-ordinated and unbalanced initially. Remember, if you have never attempted core work or ball work before, then this is a completely new way of training your body's nervous and musculoskeletal systems. It may pay to have someone like a gym instructor or friend alongside to help steady you and provide assistance until you gain balance ability and confidence. If you are at home, just position the ball near a wall so you have that added security within easy reach.

However, it is amazing how quickly your body will adapt and gain the necessary strength for you to complete the exercises. Start simple and build up slowly before progressing; definitely aim for quality before quantity.

Is it worth buying a Swiss ball?

Purchasing a Swiss ball is not expensive, and it will give you a piece of exercise equipment you can use at home before, during and after your pregnancy. Some women even like to use them: during labour; to achieve good upright posture when sitting; for leaning on; or for using as a support when squatting. Not only that, but it is also an excellent replacement chair if you have a home office or sit at a computer for any length of time, as it encourages you to maintain good ergonomic sitting posture. I am not a huge advocate of buying home exercise equipment, but this is one piece that should become well used and is well worth the moderate investment.

Baby on the ball (Fig 4.16)

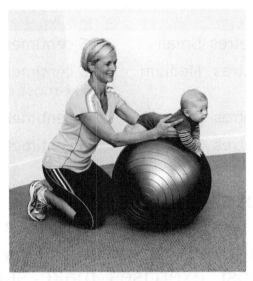

Fig.4.16

You can also use the ball as part of your baby's motor development. I put both my babies on the ball from when they were about six weeks old to encourage them to lift their heads up and strengthen their back and neck extensors—a normal developmental milestone that precedes crawling. Here's how: carefully position your baby on their tummy over the apex of the ball, forearms propped under the upper body, then gently roll them forwards and backwards, keeping a good hold of their torso as you do so. The rolling movement is a great way of stimulating their equilibrium and sensory systems. Important note: It is best to attempt this well *after* feeding time, or you and the ball may 'wear it'!

Choosing the right size Swiss ball

Height	Ball size	
Up to 145 centimetres	Small	45 centimetres (18 inches)
145–165 centimetres	Medium	55 centimetres (22 inches)—most common size
165–185 centimetres	Large	65 centimetres (26 inches)
185–195 centimetres	X-large	75 centimetres (30 inches)

Points to note

✳ When you are sitting on the ball, your bottom should not be lower than your knees.

✳ For most exercises make sure your ball is firmly inflated—a standard bike pump with an adaptor should do the trick, but some balls come with their own pump.

✳ Exceptions: Beginners may find having the ball slightly underinflated provides them with more stability on the ball initially, and a slightly softer ball is better for stretching exercises, whereas a firmer ball is better for core balance work and bouncing.

✳ Buy a burst-resistant ball, so if you do manage to puncture it, the ball will not burst but just slowly deflate.

Core exercises on the ball

What you need

Comfortable fitted clothing with your hair tied back is best for ball work, so neither gets snagged under the ball.

Sitting on ball

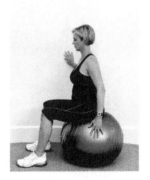

Fig.4.17

If it is your first time ever using a ball, then place it next to a wall and use one hand on the wall to steady yourself as you sit on top of the ball, feet flat on floor, about hip-distance apart (Fig.4.17). As you get used to the ball being a moveable base, take your hand off the wall and balance without support. Your abdominals, back and hip muscles will all fire up to maintain you in an upright sitting position. Play with the movement, rolling the ball a few centimetres forwards, backwards, side to side. Try a circular hip rotation in one direction and then the other. Very soon you will be at ease sitting on the ball and you will gain a good sense of your neutral spine position. (Pelvic rocking on the ball may relieve lower back ache later in pregnancy, as it gently mobilises that area.)

Sitting with foot lift

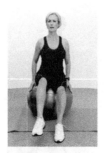

Fig.4.18

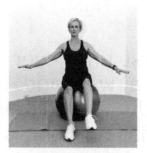

Fig.4.19

To progress, assume the upright sitting position, as above, hands resting on the sides of the ball, draw in, and brace your abdominals and lift your entire foot off the ground. Hold it for a few seconds in the air, and then lower it down to the floor again. Alternate foot lifts, right and left, holding the leg up for a few seconds, maintaining your upright sitting position and breathing evenly (Fig.4.18).

You can also try the exercise with your arms extended out either side away from the ball (Fig.4.19). If you wobble too much, drop them to the ball again. Repeat five times on each leg.

Sitting with clock arms (Figs 4.20, 4.21)

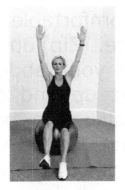

Fig.4.20

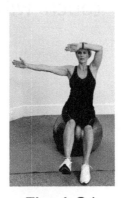

Fig.4.21

You can also experiment with using your arms to challenge your ball-sitting balance. With feet flat on floor, move both arms together over your head like the hands of clock—quarter to nine, twelve o'clock and quarter past three. Reverse the direction and repeat. Try it with alternate feet elevated off the ground. Finally, a challenging test of balance while sitting on the ball is to close your eyes and keep maintaining your position.

Ball bouncing

Once you are comfortable sitting on the ball, then add a bounce. Zip up your pelvic floor, draw in and brace your abdominals, and start bouncing your butt up and down on the ball, start off with small-range bouncing. Now, on every second bounce extend your leg and touch your toe out in front of you. Alternate heel and toe touches with each leg. As you get into a rhythm, play with adding in different leg moves; try a diagonal heel touch with alternate legs.

Hip and butt lift (not after 16 weeks of pregnancy) (Fig 4.22)

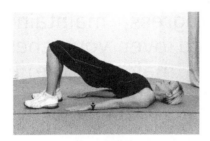

Fig.4.22

Lie on your back on the floor, feet and lower legs supported on the top of the ball, arms either side with palms down. Lift your hips up until your body forms a straight line from your toes to shoulders. Hold the position for 10–30 seconds, then release down.

Reverse bridging (Fig 4.23)

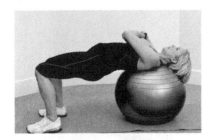

Fig.4.23

Sit on the apex of the ball, feet shoulder-width apart, and slowly walk your feet forward, letting the ball run up your back to your shoulders. Stop and elevate your hips parallel to the floor. Your head and neck rest on the ball, and your feet are flat on the floor. Maintain this position with hips lifted for 10–30 seconds. To progress, maintain the hold with your arms folded over your chest.

To progress, maintain the hip lift and lift alternate heels off the floor for a few seconds at a time (Fig 4.24).

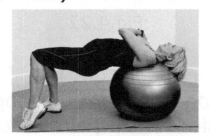

Fig.4.24

All fours balancing on top of the ball (Fig 4.25)

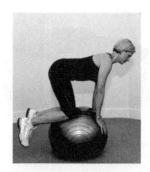

Fig.4.25

This position is suitable only during the first trimester and for those who are already familiar and comfortable with all of the above ball balancing exercises.

Stand in front of the ball, feet shoulder-width apart, and place your knees onto the front wall of the ball and both hands on top. In a rolling movement, move the ball forward and roll your body up so you are balancing on top on hands and knees. Maintain your balance on top for as long as you can, rolling back to get off the ball. Practice makes perfect with this one. Proficiency with four-point balance is the precursor to more advanced core ball balance work, like kneeling on the ball with your body upright, but remember to err on the side of caution to avoid any chance of slipping off the ball.

Key points

○ A weak core region accounts for much of the reported back pain and strain, and usually results in poor standing posture. Over time this can lead to aches, pain and injury.

○ A strong core during pregnancy is important, because toned abdominals in combination with strengthened back muscles provide your spine with stability and support. If the muscles on the front, back and sides of your spine are weak or out of balance, then your spine is a bit like a tent pole with no strong tethering ropes attached—wobbly and in danger of damage.

148

○ Modify your core exercises as your pregnancy progresses.

○ A strong core = a sturdy, stable body.

Chapter 5

The First Trimester (0–13 Weeks)

Dear Diary—Anxious Times and Eggshells

I got my first blood test result today. Tim and I were together to receive the phone call. Unlike with my first pregnancy when I was convinced I was naturally very fertile and bullet-proof, this time I am battle-worn from multiple rounds of IVF. The call from the clinic came at bang on 12.30pm as expected. 'Congratulations!' PURE SHOCK. Tears and a barely comprehensive blubbering reply to the nurse. The hCG (human chorionic gonadotrophin) levels are evidently high and that bodes well at this early stage. It's weird, with my first pregnancy getting a positive test resulted in just pure elation and excitement. This time—with the three-year IVF journey it has taken me to get to this point—it's totally different; a real mixture of anxiety and cautious excitement, with the first emotion dominating. So, it's walking on eggshells for me from now on, until I get the 'all clear' at 12 weeks.

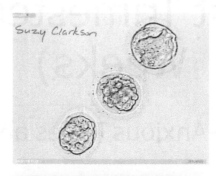

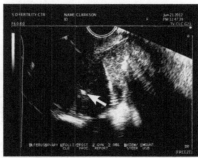

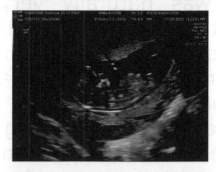

Fig.5.1 Three embryos (top) were implanted (middle, arrowed). At 12 weeks (bottom), the image of my baby can be clearly seen.

Changes afoot

Hang in there! This is a tumultuous time for your body, and it is quite likely a lot has been going on internally before you even found out you were pregnant. The fetus is growing rapidly, dividing from a cell to a bunch of cells, and then again and again. All your body's systems are on alert and are starting to adapt and make the necessary changes for this new physiological state. Hormones are surging around your body with their levels fluctuating wildly. You will probably feel some or all of these side-effects: tiredness, nausea, dizziness, stuffy nose, breathlessness and—to top it all off—you will probably feel like your bladder has the capacity of a thimble! I have one word for all of this: normal. For most women these symptoms do ease and pass, and you should feel back to the old you or close to it in your second trimester.

So why exercise now, remind me again? Because you are stimulating your placenta to grow well and you are maintaining a level of fitness that will allow you to continue on at a decent intensity when this wave of early symptoms has passed. Often exercise during the first trimester can actually decrease these unpleasant pregnancy side-effects, especially tiredness and nausea.

Exercise and side-effects

Nausea

Remember this is an annoying but normal part of early pregnancy. Following are some suggestions for helping maintain exercise despite having nausea. Try shorter bouts of exercise, 3–5 minutes, as this can often decrease the symptoms. Decrease the intensity of what you are doing—ease back and see whether you can comfortably continue. Some dietary remedies we have already looked at in Chapter 2. For example, you may find having a small snack alleviates the nausea. Some women feel so queasy when waking in the morning that they have to eat something small like a dry cracker before they get out of bed. Other possible remedies include flat soda, ginger biscuits or small, frequent meals. Although it is often called morning sickness, it can occur at any time of the day or night. Extreme early pregnancy nausea is called 'hyperemesis gravidarum'. If it causes you to regularly vomit, then make sure you drink extra fluids as you could easily become dehydrated. If you find you are suffering from this condition, it may be a reason to cut back or take a break from exercise; discuss it with your LMC.

Tiredness

Believe it or not, exercising moderately could actually alleviate your tiredness. If you find in the first trimester that you are getting particularly tired in the late afternoon and evening, then try exercising early in the day when your energy levels are less sapped, but make sure you are not overdoing it. The best way to determine this is to ascertain whether the tiredness is just sporadic and is relieved by a good night's sleep. If it is persistent tiredness verging on exhaustion, then you should decrease the intensity and duration of your exercise sessions. Once your energy levels right themselves (usually in the second trimester), you can gradually build up again and resume your regular routine. Maintaining or adding exercise to your day can also help you sleep better at night. This can help alleviate the common first trimester symptom of insomnia. You will no doubt be cutting down on, or cutting out, caffeine from your diet, and that too will help combat the wakefulness you may experience.

Dear Diary—Tiredness and Headaches

I've signed up for a free weekly reminder on the various growth stages from an online baby website – www.babycentre.co.uk I really enjoy getting their 'this week you can expect' update and seeing if I, too, am observing the changes they write about. I've had some headaches, which are very unusual for me but evidently another typical pregnancy side-effect, and bizarrely they come on during the night. I am finding I 'hit the wall' with extreme tiredness at about 9pm and just have to go to bed, but then I wake up at about 4am. I just lie there and doze, sometimes I get back to sleep but there's no point worrying about it. I tell myself that being horizontal is still restful for my body.

I am also traversing a careful balance of having enough water but not too much so I don't have to get up multiple times in the night to pee. If anything I have more fluid during the day and less in the evening, and that seems to work. I have also mastered the art of getting from bed to the toilet and back again with just one eye half-open, which almost feels as though I haven't fully woken up so I can ease back into sleep ... Although I learnt the hard and bruised way of making sure now that the en-suite sliding glass door is open before lights out.

Dizzy spells

During the first trimester, when your body is gradually getting accustomed to a change in circulatory requirements, you may experience short bouts of dizziness if you suddenly change positions, in particular when getting up from the floor. This is because your body is in the process of producing more blood and fluid, but until it gets to about the right amount (usually by the second trimester) some women will experience the symptoms of 'vascular under-fill'. It is nothing to be concerned about, but is just something to be aware of, and perhaps a reason to take large or sudden changes of movement at a slower pace.

Amount of exercise

There is no one-size-fits-all answer to how much exercise to do when it comes to exercise during pregnancy. There is no one programme or set of exercises that would be both effective and suitable for the broad range of women over the age of 35 who will pick up this book. What I can give you are basic programmes, advice and tools to have at your disposal to tailor-make your own exercise programme; one that suits both your goals and fitness level, and always keeping in mind a flexible attitude that takes into account your specific journey and how you feel day-to-day. As we discussed in Chapter 1, how much you exercise during your pregnancy is largely determined by your fitness level when you conceived. If you were fit and active already, then continuing on is highly recommended. If you were mostly sedentary without any regular exercise programme, then you should class yourself as a beginner and apply common-sense principles to gradually build up both the duration and the intensity of whatever exercise you attempt.

Guidelines

Most women in their first trimester will feel a bit off colour now and then (thank you hormones). They will notice an increase in weight—somewhere around 1.5 to 3 kilograms spread around the hip, abdomen and thigh areas (see more on this in Chapter 2).

For **previously inactive** pregnant women, it is important to gradually build up your aerobic exercise endurance. You may start with just 15 minutes of aerobic exercise three times a week. This might sound relatively little, but it is a significant and worthy start and will be something you can build on, progressing to 20–30 minutes of moderate level activity three to five days of the week.

For the pregnant **experienced exerciser,** you may wish to continue on with a regime similar to what you have been doing prior to pregnancy, but taking into account your altered state and modifying accordingly. A good rule of thumb is 40–60 minutes of exercise most (five or six) days of the week. You may find you have to modify how hard you work out if you typically exercise at a high level, but those who are used to a more moderate level will probably not have to alter intensity at all.

Tips for sticking to an exercise programme

✳ **Do it first thing** If you can, try to do your exercise first thing in the morning. Getting it out of the way at the beginning of the day means you are less likely to fob it off because of other commitments. In our family we manage this several mornings a week by me getting up and out of the house for a jog or power-walk with the dog while my husband gets the breakfast routine underway. I also utilise the kids' crèche at the gym to get my workout done early while my son is playing with other kids. It might be because I am a morning person, but every time I leave my exercise until later in the day I find I am less motivated to complete it and it runs the risk of being flicked when other more pressing matters compete for my time. I also find my mental stress levels are elevated because I know it is still one more thing I need to make time for as the hours in the day march on.

✳ **Keep an exercise diary** Use the template shown in Chapter 1, or simply note in your diary or smartphone what you have done each day. It's a record that quickly becomes a motivating tool for you to look back on and celebrate your achievements each week. It is also a good idea to show your LMC at your regular check-ups so that they get the full picture of what you are doing on your pregnancy journey.

✳ **Success in numbers** Exercising with a group or with another person of a similar age or stage increases your adherence to a regular regime. Again, you are less likely not to do it if you have made the effort to get to a class at a gym or you are meeting a friend to power-walk or jog. Motivating music from a group session or a motivating chat with a friend makes exercising fun, and if it is fun you will stick with it.

✳ **If it's fun, it's fine** It may sound twee, but there also has to be a fun element to your workouts. Trying to exercise regularly by doing an activity that you passionately dislike just won't work. What you choose to do needs to be attractive to you; that way, you will stick with it. For example, I have never been that keen on swimming lengths. I don't mind being in water, but it's just not been one of those activities I have gravitated towards. Even knowing that swimming is a good activity to do during pregnancy didn't get me jumping in initially; however, during the latter half of my first pregnancy, I really enjoyed aqua jogging and went to the local indoor pool for regular sessions. Sometimes I was able to persuade friends to join me with the promise of a good chat while doing the exercise and a café stop afterwards! It was a lovely sensation having my heavy pregnant belly supported by the buoyancy of the water while still being able to get a good cardiovascular workout. We'll explore aqua jogging in more detail later, but the point is 'do something you enjoy' and keep your mind open to try new things. Variety is the spice of life. It will help you stick to your exercise programme and get results.

What to wear to exercise

Your breasts will naturally become fuller over the course of the pregnancy in preparation for breastfeeding. Many women experience breast changes right from early pregnancy, with swelling and tenderness tending to be the most common symptoms. Pregnant or not, it is always a good idea to wear a workout bra that gives good support and minimises bounce or stretching of the delicate breast tissue. Even in the first trimester you may need to be refitted for a workout bra, and you may find you need several more fittings until you reach full term. Having a good bra that fits minimises or eliminates breast discomfort when you are doing exercise that involves jumping up and down, such as jogging or aerobic classes. You may also find that your breasts are so tender that it is uncomfortable to lie down on your stomach. I have found that for jogging, in particular, wearing two workout bras gives the best support: underneath, wear a comfortable full-cup support workout bra, and over the top of that a close-fitting workout tank-top. This seems to really minimise uncomfortable 'bounce'.

The only other major consideration with workout clothing is to dress in layers so that, as you build up heat from your exercising, you can peel off a layer and cool down without doing a full striptease! A cotton lycra pair of workout tights or pants with a wide stretchy waistband, preferably adjustable, is also a good investment for your ever-expanding girth.

Dear Diary—Boobs

Okay, this is ridiculous: I've gone from a 12B to a 12DD—and I'm still expanding. Last pregnancy I reached a 12F, which according to hubby was 'impressive' but useless as he wasn't allowed near them! I'm just not used to big boobs. For me they are foreign appendages that have a life and gravity of their own, which means they are mostly pendulous and sore. I've had to get new bras.

Odours of strong foods really turn my stomach now. Onions or mushrooms cooking have me running from the room, and there's a scented room diffuser that I used to love that I've had to throw out as it makes me feel sick.

I'm balancing the demands of being at work with the walking I am doing, and if I think I'm pushing it I just back off. My daily nausea doesn't seem to be abating. I'm not actually being sick, but I'm off my food. I'm still on decaf coffee as I have been for the years of IVF attempts, and I'm being very careful about making sure I only eat 'pregnancy-safe' foods. So long sushi, I'll see you in seven months or so!

The essential elements

We've already discussed how pregnancy is not the time to take on physical challenges like training for an event or competition. Most mums-to-be have one or more of these goals:

weight control, fitness, fun, wellbeing, strength, injury prevention and posture maintenance. A balanced exercise regime that covers these sorts of goals is one which incorporates three vital elements.

1. **cardiovascular fitness**—sweaty exercise that stimulates your heart and lungs
2. **strength training**—working against resistance to keep your muscles strong
3. **flexibility**—stretching for good posture and prevention of injury.

Let's look at what you can do in each domain.

Cardiovascular exercise

Research concludes that regular sustained 'weight-bearing exercise' is the best type for pregnant women because it clearly complements the adaptations to pregnancy, but it is important to get the frequency and intensity right.

What to do

Gym-based aerobic-type classes are a good form of cardiovascular exercise during the first trimester, and you shouldn't have to modify too many of the moves. If you have already been running or jogging, you can continue on with your usual regime. If you are just beginning this type of impact exercise, then build up gradually from power-walking to a combination of walking and jogging, and level off at about 30 minutes of jogging, remembering to keep your effort level at 'somewhat hard' on the perceived exertion scale, or use the talk test method of monitoring intensity (see Chapter 1).

Now is a good time to introduce a type of cardiovascular fitness that you can continue with through your second and third trimesters and right up to term. For example, if you are a runner or jogger then you may like to get familiar with a low-impact form of cardiovascular exercise on a stationary machine – such as a stepper, a cross-trainer or a stationary bike. Getting familiar with these sorts of machines (which are most commonly found at gyms) will give you more options for exercise as your pregnancy progresses.

Avoid increasing the amount of exercise

Limit the stress of upping your exercise demands during the first trimester. However, if you want to increase the amount of cardiovascular type exercise, then restrict it to no more than an extra 30 minutes a week. Again, a reminder: this is not the time to train hard or subject yourself to intense exercise endeavours. Nor is it a time to exercise to lose weight or to stop yourself from changing shape.

Warming up and cooling down

Warming up and cooling down are safe physiological practices that apply to exercising regardless of whether you are pregnant or not, but since you are, it is even more important as your heart rate and blood pressure are more prone to fluctuate. Warming up gently eases your heart and lungs into coping with the increased demands for oxygen that accompany activity, plus it minimises the risk of muscle or ligament injury and allows you to get the most out of your workout. The average person who spends 30 to 60 minutes exercising at moderate intensity should spend 5 to 10 minutes warming up and the same time cooling down.

Consider which major muscles you will be using during your exercise session, and warm them up with a gentle version of the activity. For jogging, walk briskly to warm up. For tennis, jog a little, move your shoulders in circles and hit the ball gently. For weight-lifting, warm up and do mobility exercises for the muscles you will be using. Do a lightly weighted first set, and then for your actual workout those particular muscle fibres required to work hard will be ready for heavier weights. The harder and longer you intend to work out, the longer and more thorough your warm-up and cool-down need to be.

The ahhhhh factor

Something I readily admit is that I love the cool-down time, especially if I have challenged myself during the workout. It feels good and it is physiologically advantageous to taper off rather than stop exercising immediately. A cool-down slows your circulation, and brings your body temperature and heart rate back to normal. This process often takes a little longer when you are pregnant, hence the importance of easing off gently. Allow at least five minutes for your cool-down. If you cool down properly you won't feel dizzy when you get in the shower after your workout.

Dear Diary—7 weeks and counting

I evidently now have a uterus the size of a grapefruit; it has grown in size from the pre-pregnancy dimension of a clenched fist. The only symptoms I have so far are tender boobs which have ballooned and some niggling nausea. Both symptoms I'm actually welcoming as it means I am still on-track. To be honest, given the rocky road to get to this point I think I'd accept any symptoms without complaining. Which is just as well, as I'm having daily intramuscular injections (part of the IVF regime) to keep my levels of progesterone on-track. They're not pleasant and, given that they have to go quite deep into the muscle, I get hubby to do them as there's no way I could plunge a needle in that far. I now am sporting a 'numb lumpy bum'. Where the injection sites are, it's numb to the touch and quite lumpy, despite me massaging it. Once I get past my eight-week scan, then the embryo is officially called a fetus, that's when the critical organs are forming. I am taking my pregnancy vitamins fastidiously, especially daily folic acid. Fingers crossed for the next scan results.

Suitable first-trimester cardiovascular exercise

√ **Walking** A great beginner exercise and *the* exercise for during and after pregnancy. It is cheap, requires little skill and you can do it pretty much anywhere, any time. The key with walking is to have good supportive shoes, and choose a route that is suitable for your current fitness level. Beginners should be mostly on flat ground; those more advanced can incorporate hills and inclines. Take some water with you if possible, swing your arms, be aware of your core muscles, and brace your abdominals. You can even do a set of pelvic floor exercises while on the move! The terrain and your speed will determine the intensity of your walking workout. During your first trimester you should aim to be puffing a little, with a glow to your cheeks after your walk. Remember, if it is a walk for the purpose of exercising, then *get moving.* A stroll is not a fitness-promoting walk. It gets you out and about, yes, but if you want the health benefits from cardiovascular exercise then pick up the pace and make your walk brisk.

√ **Jogging/Running** It is not a time to begin running, but if you are a regular runner then you can continue on. Warm up and cool down adequately – 5–10 minutes each. Avoid running down hills as this may provide extra strain on your joints, but if this is unavoidable, then keep your knees soft to allow for as much cushioning of the impact as possible. Be careful with running uphill, as your heart rate will elevate quickly. Consider a run/walk combo where you run on the flat and walk up steep hills. Take water with you and keep hydrated. If it's warm weather, have layers of clothing to peel off or modify your intensity so you avoid getting too hot.

√ **Cycling** If you have not cycled before becoming pregnant, it is probably not the best choice of exercise to take up now; choose to exercise on a stationary cycle instead. If you are familiar with bike riding, just be aware of not putting yourself in a situation where you might have a fall or take a tumble. Now is definitely not the time to take up mountain-bike riding!

Home-based and gym cardio equipment

Often personal preference determines the sort of equipment you feel most comfortable on. You can try a cardio workout that utilises several different pieces of equipment; spending 10–15 minutes on each with short changeover times in between can combat the potential boredom of using just one machine.

√ **Stationary bike** A good beginner exercise, make sure the seat height is adjusted so that there is still about a 10° bend in your knee when your leg is extended at the bottom of the pedal circle. You can also use a recumbent bike with the same knee-angle to get the right leg length. You will need to work a little harder to achieve the same intensity of exercise in the recumbent position as your body weight is more supported in this position.

√ **Elliptical trainer** This machine requires reasonable balance, but its motion is low-impact and mimics functional forward movement. It also uses arms and leg movements together (if you are on a machine that has moveable arms), so this will raise your heart rate more quickly than other cardio machines.

✓ **Stepper** These are good for legs, buttocks and back strength. Make sure you maintain good upright posture, and if you are unsure of how to use the machine, get a gym instructor to give you some tips on good positioning and how to adjust the resistance.

✓ **Rower** If you are a beginner to rowing, make sure you get someone to show you correct technique as it is not just a case of pulling the row bar and straightening your legs. Well it is, but in a particular way, as it is all down to timing, making sure the large leg muscles are the powerhouses that generate the movement. Press your shoulders down and avoid hunching over with your upper body. Switch on your core abdominal muscles to give extra support to your lower back.

✓ **Treadmill** A good piece of equipment for beginners, as it is adaptable to all fitness levels by adjusting both intensity and gradient. It works legs and buttocks and is a very functional activity. And the bonus: it can be done in any sort of weather and even with a friend on a machine alongside for moral support and chatting.

Water-supported exercise

Any water-supported exercise gets a BIG TICK during pregnancy and is a firm favourite of many women. You will find it increasingly useful the further through your pregnancy you are, especially in the second and third trimesters when you are carrying a lot more baby weight. The water will also dissipate any body heat built up during exercise, so there is less chance of overheating. Check that the pool temperature is in the range of about 27–30° Celsius—there should be a pool temperature gauge displayed. It is always a good idea to shower off after a pool workout to wash off any chlorine or pool chemicals.

✓ **Swimming** Open to any fitness level, this is a low-risk, ideal allover workout. Even if you are a beginner, you can get in and get going without too much fussing about. It is great aerobic exercise if you can manage at least a few lengths in a row; the more the merrier. There is no bumping or jarring, unless you hit the end of the pool or another swimmer! If you were a regular swimmer before becoming pregnant, then the normal aerobic exercise guidelines apply of 30–60 minutes at moderate intensity.

✓ **Aqua jogging** Either you can do this in chest- or shoulder-depth water and just jog along the pool floor using your arms and legs, or you can do it in deep water with the use of a floatation device. Aqua jogging in deep water is often used by runners for rehabilitating after an injury; it is essentially running but without the impact. The floatation vest (often provided by the facility) straps firmly around your torso, helping to keep you in the upright position. Pump your arms as if you were running normally and keep your fingers together. Try experimenting with flat-blade hand positions to get more or less resistance from the water as you jog along. Lifting your knees higher creates a bigger movement and more water resistance which will elevate your heart rate. Even when jogging along at a decent speed and with a good range of movement you still should be able to conduct a conversation, so invite a friend to keep you company. Beginners start with a 5–10-minute session and build up from there. If you are reasonably fit, be aware that you need to keep up the pace and range of motion, as coasting is easy and you are only cheating yourself!

✓ **Aqua aerobics** You can join in an aqua aerobics class at any stage of your pregnancy, just make sure that after the first trimester you mention you are pregnant to the instructor. Some facilities may even run specific pregnancy aqua aerobics classes. Most classes will involve using the water to provide resistance to your movements, and have the usual class structure of warm-up, exercise session, and then cool-down and stretching. Don't overdo it: watch for feeling dizzy or light-headed, and if you experience these symptoms get to the edge of the pool and take a break or conclude your workout.

Group fitness classes

Group fitness classes are motivating and give you good social contact. The fact that classes are timetabled means you make 'an appointment' in your day to exercise, and are thus less likely to forego it. However, this is not the time to take up high-impact aerobics, boxing or combat-type sessions, but less intense classes should be suitable. Tell the instructor you are pregnant and that you would like suitable modifications to moves offered throughout. If you have not participated in classes previously, then you may wish to start with walking, swimming or using stationary cardio machines to get low-risk but sufficient base aerobic conditioning exercise. If you have regularly attended classes, then the first trimester should not involve too many modifications. Your RPE (recommended perceived exertion level) should be around 6–7.

In this section I outline pregnancy modifications for a variety of Les Mills classes as their group fitness programme is available in 80 countries worldwide, but of course they are not the only class options. There are many other suitable exercise classes you can attend at gyms and in the local community. If the class you choose to attend is similar in content to those outlined here then cast your eye over the modifications and adapt as necessary. As a general rule, for any class you should always let the instructor know you are pregnant so they can provide additional cueing and offer alternative movements that are more suitable for pregnancy. If you feel the instructor does not have the knowledge to modify the movements accordingly, then use your own sensible judgement and always err on the side of caution. Do less rather than more.

✓ **Cycle classes** These low-impact classes can provide quite intense aerobic exercise, but the pedal resistance you set on your bike is under your control and therefore as a form of training these classes are useful for all three trimesters (with modifications). If you are a beginner, ask for plenty of advice on setting up the bike correctly for your height and size; most are widely adjustable. Do a beginners class or an introduction class to see if it is your thing. Most bikes also have the option of cycle shoes that have cleats on the bottom that click into the pedal, or toe baskets that fit normal gym shoes. For those experienced cycle class attendees, the only modification you should need to make in the first trimester is to keep your heart rate to a moderate 140–160 beats per minute, or an RPE of 6–7.

✓ **Aerobic/Step classes** This type of class is generally fine during the first trimester. Towards the latter half of this trimester you may wish to lower the level of your step and limit twisting movements. BODYVIVE™ (a Les Mills group fitness programme) is low-impact cardio fitness, functional strength training and flexibility work, so a good option.

✓ **Kick-boxing/Cross-fit classes** These are classified as extreme conditioning options, and are not recommended during pregnancy.

✓ **Mixed martial arts classes** This style of class—like Les Mills's COMBAT™—is not recommended to begin during pregnancy, but if you are already a class participant then drop your intensity by about a third and take particular care with twisting movements.

✓ **Circuit classes** These involve aerobic moves interspersed with exercising on machines in a class format, and are not recommended to begin during pregnancy. For regular participants, decrease the intensity so that your heart rate stays roughly between 140–160 beats per minute.

✓ **Other combination class examples** BODYBALANCE™ (a Les Mills group fitness programme) is a good low-impact choice during pregnancy, as it emphasises stretching, core strengthening and relaxation. It began as a combination of pilates, yoga and t'ai chi-type moves, but has evolved into its own flowing style and format which is ideal (with modifications) for all stages of pregnancy. During the first trimester you will not have to alter any moves. As part of a balanced fitness programme you may find that this sort of class provides a good opportunity for valuable stretching and rejuvenating relaxation. CXWORX™ (a Les Mills group fitness programme) is a short 30-minute workout that focuses on core and functional strengthening (abdominals and butt). It is suitable for the first trimester.

Interval training

Interval training is a concept that can be applied to most forms of cardiovascular exercise. It basically means alternating between going faster for a set time at a particular activity and then slowing down for a period of time to allow some recovery; for example, running for 2 minutes then walking for 4 minutes. In principle, interval training is good to add variety to any cardiovascular workout, but as it is a reasonably intense form of training (often used to help overcome a fitness training plateau), it is probably better attempted when you are not pregnant.

Strength training

Strength training, resistance training and weight training are all terms that essentially mean the same thing: you are pushing or pulling against a resistance that requires effort by your body's musculature. This type of training is great during pregnancy as it helps you maintain strength to support your growing body weight, builds muscle tone (firmness) and allows you to regain your figure faster after giving birth. As with all forms of exercise undertaken during pregnancy, make sure you discuss your intentions with your LMC.

Strength training is beneficial to women whether pregnant or not, as from about 25 years on the muscle content in your body naturally begins a slow process of atrophy (wasting away) at a rate of about 228 grams (that's roughly half a block of butter) a year *unless* you maintain it by exercising—hence the saying 'use it or lose it'. Of course non-exercisers may not notice this change as the muscle content will most likely be replaced by fat, meaning they may *look* roughly the same. But where it is noticeable is in body composition and corresponding metabolism. Muscle tissue is energy-hungry; it requires calories to exist. Fat does not; it is essentially dormant, sitting there, along for the ride. An increase in the amount of lean muscle tissue in your body means you become a better fat-burning machine.

Whatever type of 'resistance' you choose to use—your own body weight, balancing on a Swiss ball, working with free weights or machines or stretchy bands or cables—it will help maintain lean muscle mass and improve your strength and endurance. Resistance training shapes and firms up your body better than any other form of exercise. Often women shy away from strength training, believing incorrectly that they will 'bulk up'. The reality is that bulking up is very difficult to achieve for women and requires a nutritional programme dedicated to weight gain in combination with lifting extremely heavy weights and many hours of training. Many women find that if they add some regular strength training to their fitness regime they notice a big improvement in their body composition—less fat, more firmness. Another advantage of strength training is that it helps increase bone density which is important for the prevention of osteoporosis (brittle bone disease). If you are keen to achieve a feminine but fit-looking physique, then stick to high repetition and low to moderate weights which will help you achieve a look of definition and firmness.

During pregnancy strength training is a very effective and time-efficient way to exercise, so in an ideal world you would aim for two or three sessions a week, working every major muscle group, in addition to cardiovascular training. During your first trimester there is very little that needs to be modified. Basic principles apply: it's not a time to increase your weights; don't overexert yourself or work to failure; keep your movements controlled and smooth; avoid excess range of movement; keep cool and hydrated; breathe evenly throughout the exercises; and work at moderate intensity. Maintain good alignment throughout your exercises, be aware of your posture, and use a neutral spine stance for standing exercises, brace your abdominals and zip up your pelvic floor. Be particularly vigilant about not holding your breath when exercising. A handy phrase to remember is: *exhale on exertion.*

Towards the end of the first trimester you can start focusing on those muscles that will serve you particularly well as your baby bump grows and your shape changes: toned gluteal or buttock muscles will help with pelvic stability, and of course strong deep abdominals and back muscles will provide support for the spine. It is also worth considering upper-body strengthening to help with good posture and to gain functional strength for the increased lifting and carrying you will be doing with a newborn baby.

If you are beginning a resistance or weights programme during your first trimester, you should keep the weights light and the repetitions high. If you have already been doing a regular weights workout, you can continue on with your usual programme, regarding the first trimester as a weights 'maintenance' phase and not increasing your loads, repetitions or sets. Allow 24 hours between strength-training sessions to provide sufficient recovery. Abdominal strengthening during the first trimester will not require much, if any, modification. The baby is tiny and growing within the pelvic region, so any sort of abdominal exercises are generally fine to undertake up to 12 weeks' gestation. This is a good time to get those deep abdominal muscles strong (transverse abdominis—TVA) so that they provide good core support. If you are new to exercising and abdominal exercises, then focus predominantly on strengthening the deep abdominals and pelvic tilting.

Strength classes

You can participate in group resistance classes like Les Mills's BODYPUMP™. This is like other gym classes to music, except the focus is not on bouncing around but instead on toning the muscles by using a barbell or weighted plates in a group environment. It works on the basis of high repetitions and low load to tone and condition the entire body. The benefits of a BODYPUMP™ class are that it's basically a supervised weights session, but jazzed up to motivating music. You can alter the weights to suit your level of fitness, and, because you are under the instructor's experienced eye, you are more likely to make sure your technique is correct and put in a good effort. If you are a regular participant, keep your weights at your usual level or decrease slightly; if you are a beginner, use one of the smallest weights available and concentrate on technique. As your pregnancy progresses it is advisable to let the instructor know that you are pregnant, as they will be able to provide verbal cues for suitable weight levels and alternative options for exercises and positioning.

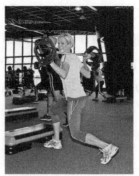

Own strength-training programme

You can continue with your own gym weights programme if you have been doing so prior to getting pregnant, or you can get a qualified gym instructor or personal trainer to prepare a programme for you, making sure you tell them that you are pregnant.

The major muscle groups are: gluteals (buttocks); quadriceps (front thigh); hamstrings (back of thigh); latissimus dorsi (lateral, upper and mid-back); erector spinae (central back); rhomboids (central upper back); pectorals (chest); deltoids (shoulders); triceps (back upper arm); biceps (front upper arm); gastrocnemius, soleus (calf); obliques; rectus abdominis; and transverse abdominis (abdominals).

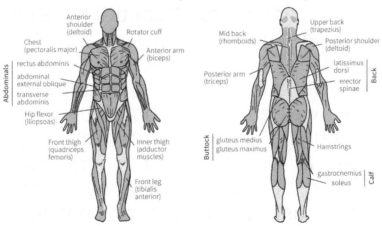

Fig.5.1 Muscles of the body

You may choose to use weight training machines in a gym environment, although as you are usually sitting or supported by the machine and isolating specific muscles, this is not as functional as using free weights, barbells, dumbbells, or a Swiss ball which encourages more core stabilisation.

A full body routine suitable for gym-based strength training during the first trimester

Reps and sets

A number of repetitions (reps) of an exercise—for example 5, 10 or 15—make up a set. During this stage of pregnancy, aim for approximately 15 repetitions (anywhere from 10–20), and 2–3 sets of each exercise, resting between sets for about 30–60 seconds. You can lower the sets and reps for the subsequent trimesters. Repetitions should be performed in a slow, controlled manner. As a general guide to the speed of movement involved, it should take 2–3 seconds to lift or push the weight, and about the same or slightly longer to lower or release. Good technique is important for getting great results. Also, if you are in a gym and there are mirrors, use them: they are not just there to make the room look bigger, they provide excellent feedback for checking your alignment and form. After a warm-up, start with exercises for the larger muscle groups and then move on to the smaller muscles. Don't feel you need to do any exercise 'to failure' (a technique often used in weight training where someone helps you to complete the final few repetitions) as you should not be pushing this hard during pregnancy. As your pregnancy progresses, reduce the amount of weight you are using.

1 Squats

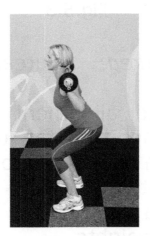

Fig.5.2

Muscles worked: gluteals, legs, core stabilisers.

These are suitable, so long as you do not have problems with your pelvis, spine or knees. Squats can be done with or without weights, and you can use a bar behind your neck or dumbbells for first trimester. Check your alignment, switch on the core, and tilt at your hips but keep your back straight.

2 Lunges

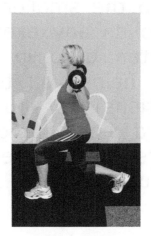

Fig.5.3

Muscles worked: gluteals, legs, core stabilisers.

Technique and alignment of the hip and knee are very important for lunging. Bend the front knee to an angle of no more than 90° with a wide split-leg stance. During the first trimester moving and static lunges are fine, with or without weights.

3 Clean and press

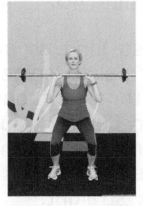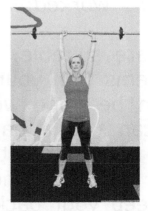

Fig.5.4

Muscles worked: shoulder girdle.

Use a barbell or dumbbells. Check your technique, smooth controlled movement, and even breathing.

4 Chest-press

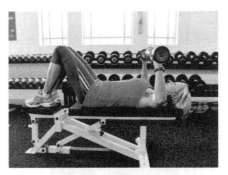

Fig.5.5

Muscles worked: pectoralis major, triceps.

Lying flat on a bench is fine for the first trimester. You can also do floor press-ups, half or full.

5 Lat pull-down

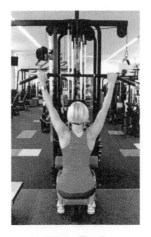

Fig.5.6

Muscles worked: latissimus dorsi.

Avoid taking the bar behind your neck. Pull it down in front of your chin, and use core stabilisers to maintain erect upper body posture.

6 Bent-over row

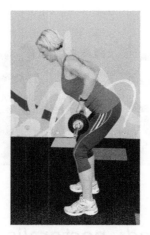

Fig.5.7

Muscles worked: mid-back, rhomboids.

Brace your abdominals, keep the back straight, and squeeze your shoulder blades together.

7 Tricep push-downs

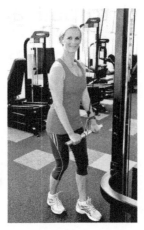

Fig.5.8

Muscles worked: long and short head of triceps.

Avoid arching your back, and use a neutral spine stance in standing.

8 Bicep curls

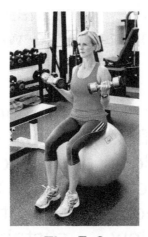

Fig.5.9

Muscles worked: biceps, forearms.

Use a barbell or dumbbells, and you could sit on a Swiss ball to add a core stabilisation element.

9 Abdominals

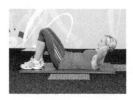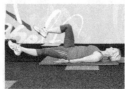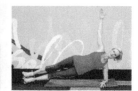

Fig.5.10

Muscles worked: rectus, obliques, deep transverse.

Three exercises: sit ups: lying with alternate leg lowering; and side static plank-holds.

Flexibility

Whether you're pregnant or not, the stretching part of a three-way exercise plan (cardiovascular, strength and flexibility components) is often the one that gets short-changed or left out completely. I have been guilty of finishing an exercise session looking at the clock and quickly tossing in a few cursory stretches when I know I would be far better served by allocating a good 10 minutes of slow, sustained stretching. Maintaining or gaining a good level of flexibility will enhance your posture, reduce your chance of injury, reduce muscle soreness, and increase the range of motion of your joints. The muscle relaxation that comes from stretching improves the circulation in your body. This allows more nutrients to get to your muscles via the blood. It prevents toxins building up and keeps tiredness at bay. Stretching is a great rejuvenator and adds to an overall feeling of relaxation and wellbeing.

When you stretch you are not only lengthening the muscles, you are also attempting to maintain range in the connective tissues in and around them. The resistance you feel when you get into a stretch position is both tight muscles as well as connective tissue, and that is why it is important to hold each stretch for a decent length of time—up to 30 seconds. Muscles release relatively quickly compared to tough connective tissue, which benefits from more sustained stretching (but within the usual range).

The aim of stretching is to maintain a balance between equal and opposite muscle groups. It is useful for chronically tight areas, such as the hamstrings, calves, back of the neck, front of the shoulder and lower back. For overall body balance, your aim should be to stretch the tight muscles and strengthen the weak ones. The best time to stretch is after warming up and after cooling down.

Extra stretchiness in pregnancy

During pregnancy your body produces a range of hormones, but the crucial one in terms of flexibility is relaxin, which by its very name hints at what it does. Its purpose is to gradually increase joint laxity (looseness) so that during the birth process there is more 'give' from the ligaments and tendons of the pelvis to allow the baby's passage down and through. However, relaxin does not act only on the pelvis, and it can tend to make ligaments, tendons and the joints they support throughout the entire body more flexible. The current guidelines therefore recommend 'moderate' stretching and not pushing your stretching beyond what is a normal range of movement for you.

As your pregnancy progresses you should also decrease the length of time you hold a stretch position. A sensible approach is to stick to your normal range of movement when stretching and don't be tempted to push beyond that. If you are attending yoga, Pilates or specific stretching classes, then advise the instructor of your pregnancy and they should adapt the positions for you as required and give you safe stretching options. If the person taking the class is not knowledgeable about appropriate modifications for pregnancy, then it is probably best to seek out a specific pregnancy yoga or Pilates session. From the second trimester onwards, it is not sufficient for the instructor to just tell you to 'take it easy' or 'do what you can'.

Stretches to avoid

The advice to avoid the supine position (lying on your back) for any length of time applies to part way through your second trimester (after 16 weeks) and is due to pressure from the expanded uterus pushing down on the major blood vessels potentially obstructing flow which could leave you dizzy or light headed. During the first trimester this is not considered a problem. There is no reason to exclude any stretching position at this stage.

Safe workout structure

Warm up incorporating light mobility stretches, follow with the workout component, then cool down incorporating longer, relaxing stretches. It is important to warm up before you stretch. This prevents injury, because a supple body bends more easily than a rigid one. You will also get the maximum benefit from your stretches. Think of a muscle as a piece of chewing gum: it will snap if you stretch it when it is cold. Warm up the muscles and they respond and function better. The sort of stretching to do as part of your warm-up is large muscle movements, such as circling your arms, gently rotating the spine side to side, lifting your knee into your chest. Towards the end of your exercise session is the best time for performing sustained static stretch positions.

Fig.5.11 Stretches for the main muscle groups

The perfect stretch

Ease gently into a stretch, making sure you maintain correct alignment. Don't bounce when stretching as this can tighten the muscle rather than loosen it. Stretch until you feel a mild to moderate tension, relax, exhale and hold the position for 10–30 seconds. You should not feel any pain. You may feel the initial tension in the muscle easing off as you hold the stretch – this is the muscle 'letting go'. Repeat each stretch 2–3 times, breathing deeply and evenly.

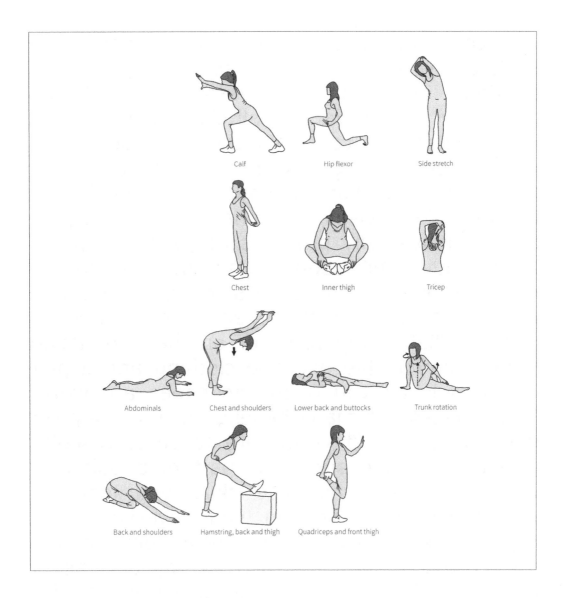

Calf   Hip flexor   Side stretch

Chest   Inner thigh   Tricep

Abdominals   Chest and shoulders   Lower back and buttocks   Trunk rotation

Back and shoulders   Hamstring, back and thigh   Quadriceps and front thigh

Pilates

Pilates is a form of exercise that improves flexibility and strength and aims to create a balance in the body with its core focus on ideal posture and trunk stability. Strengthening the pelvic floor, deep abdominals and reinforcement of an effective deep breathing technique are key components of Pilates, all of which are particularly useful during pregnancy. Pilates sessions are typically one-on-one with an instructor or with very small class sizes (5–10), so modifications can be made to ensure it is an appropriate activity throughout all three trimesters. You work at your own level though a series of exercises, with the instructor helping you to individually progress at your own pace. Most studios will require you to do a private consultation first and then sign up for a series of classes. The exercises are done either on specific Pilates apparatus or on the floor using mats. Comfortable exercise clothing and a pair of socks is all you need; no shoes are worn. While Pilates has many benefits for the pregnant woman, it doesn't contribute to cardiovascular fitness, so make sure it is part of a balanced exercise programme. The skills you learn in Pilates can help you in your everyday life, especially with good posture, movement patterns and correct lifting. This activity will also be of great benefit to you during delivery and for getting your body back into shape after birth.

Considerations for the first trimester

If you are new to Pilates, look for a beginner class and advise the instructor of your pregnancy. You should be able to participate in all of the moves during the first trimester, but of course listen to your body and ask the instructor for modifications if you need to. Often classes can be only as good as the instructor, so seek out a good teacher—ask around for recommendations.

Yoga

Whether you are new to yoga or already an experienced yogi, you can enjoy the benefits of this form of exercise while pregnant. Yoga is a form of exercise that unites both the body and mind through positions (or asanas) that enhance strength, flexibility and relaxation. It transcends purely physical fitness with its emphasis also on breathing and meditation techniques. Many women find yoga a rewarding activity to do during pregnancy, as it can be adjusted to any fitness level and provides valuable stress relief.

There are many different types of yoga—Hatha, Iyengar, Ashtanga and Bikram are the most typical forms practised in the Western world. Some forms are more intense than others, and Bikram in particular is conducted in a hot environment. *While you are pregnant do not do Bikram yoga, as it is important to avoid overheating.* It is also wise to avoid the more dynamic styles from the second trimester on, or at the very least make sure you have an instructor who is specifically trained in modifications for pregnancy.

There are many synergies with yoga and pregnancy. Yoga teaches you to listen to your body, which is a valuable skill throughout your pregnancy. Yoga has a strong focus on the breath, and teaches you how to breathe calmly and deeply—this is particularly valuable both as a general relaxation technique and also during labour. Yoga teaches you how to focus and calm the mind; again, this can be of huge benefit to you during the early stages of the birth process. Using both breathing and relaxation techniques may mean you can diminish the amount of pain you feel and possibly even lessen the amount of pain relief used during labour.

If you are beginning yoga for the first time during this trimester, either seek out a beginner level class or a prenatal session, and always advise the instructor of your pregnancy, particularly if your physical shape does not reveal your new state. During the first trimester you should be able to do most yoga moves, but common sense applies: if a pose feels wrong, skip it or seek advice on how to adjust to a position where you feel more comfortable. If you were a regular yoga attendee prior to becoming pregnant, then continue on with your usual practice (except Bikram—see the earlier cautionary advice), although you may choose to decrease the intensity or start to incorporate some pregnancy adaptations into your routine.

Dear Diary—Gums and 'Staying Mum'

My gums have been bleeding a little bit; nothing major, but I've noticed it and I'm sure it's not because I've just got over-zealous with brushing. Again according to the books it's another pregnancy idiosyncrasy. I'm still not showing a bump yet, though I've thickened up around my waist. I've told a limited number of people about my pregnancy so far, just a handful of close friends and family, as I don't want to tempt fate. I wonder if the phrase 'staying mum about things' comes from this sort of situation? Anyway that's what I'm doing—'staying mum'. My doctor reckons that, because of the trials and tribulations I've been through to get to this point, my anxiety over things potentially going wrong will stay for the entire pregnancy and I won't be truly placated until I have an actual baby in my arms. Great!

Two home workouts

Each of these workouts is suitable for the first trimester, and each is of approximately

50–60 minutes' duration. The first is a purely muscle toning workout covering all the main muscle groups. The second is a cross-training workout, incorporating a combination of cardiovascular exercise with some strength training and stretching.

Remember that variety is the key, so intersperse these workouts at home with other activities that you enjoy. See the options above for other cardiovascular exercise or group fitness classes.

What you will need

Space
An area to work out in of about 2 metres square. If it's fine weather you might want to consider doing some of the exercises outside.

Equipment
A towel or a mat. I recommend buying a stretchy band or flex band to provide some resistance for strength training. The bands are made of rubber, so keep them out of direct sunlight to preserve their integrity. They are not expensive and can be purchased at sporting goods stores or online. They come in different sizes and resistance levels; you may wish to purchase a couple to have both a light and a medium resistance. Some designs are tubing that has adjustable handles so you can alter length. This sort of equipment is a great tool

for home workouts; they are easy to use and very portable. Other names that the bands are sold under include latex resistance, aerobic bands or resistance tubes.

Workout 1: Toning at home

With each exercise: remember to zip up your pelvic floor muscles and brace your abdominals to provide good lower back support and strong core stabilisation throughout.

Beginner level: 1 set of each exercise (after 2–3 sessions you can increase to 2 and then 3 sets).

Previously active and fit prior to pregnancy: 2–3 sets, completing each exercise in a slow and controlled manner so you feel the exertion but not exhaustion.

1 Intensity squats

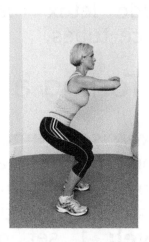

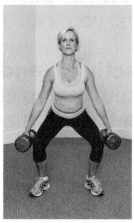

Fig.5.12

Muscles used: Front and back of thigh, butt and back. An added bonus to this exercise is that it strengthens the muscles often used in labour. The squatting position opens up the pelvic area an extra 10%. It makes sense to strengthen the muscles that are required now for squatting as it may make your job a little easier if you choose to give birth in a squat position. Older mums who have not been very physically active in recent years will really benefit from this exercise, as later you will always be bobbing up and down, picking up your baby from the floor, not to mention the toys and all the other paraphernalia that come with a new child in the household. The squat must be performed with precision, and the slower the better. Consciously think of squeezing and tightening your buttocks when you rise up each time.

Key points: Feet slightly wider than hip-distance apart. Bend at the knees and hips. Keep your back straight and tilt forward slightly at the hips as if going to sit down on a chair. Squat until thighs are no lower than parallel to floor, pause briefly at this lowered position, perform 5 small range bounces, then smoothly lift back up again. When down in the squat position, check the alignment of your knees: they should point in line with the toes but not extend beyond them. Turn toes out more to target inner thighs. This exercise can be performed with just body weight as the small bounces at the base will really increase the load on the leg muscles. You can also add dumbbells or a barbell if you prefer.

1 set: 20 repetitions. Lower for 2, small range bounce in lower position for 5 counts, slowly rise.

Beginners – 1 set.

Advanced – 2–3 sets.

2 Lunges

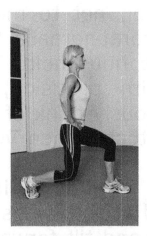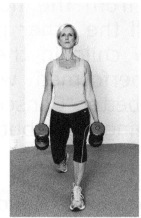

Fig.5.13

Muscles used: legs, butt, back and core. Lunges are a very functional activity; consider how often you lunge forward or bend down to pick something up off the floor.

Key points: On a flat surface, with good supportive shoes and feet parallel, hip-distance apart, take an extra-long step forward with one leg and bend the front knee to about 90°. Your hands should be on your hips or extended out either side for balance. Tuck your tailbone under. Lower your body vertically by bending the back knee down towards the ground. Rise up again to standing position, pressing down hard through the heel of your front leg. Keep your shoulders back and the entire movement smooth and controlled. Remember to drop down without any forward movement, to avoid over-stressing the front knee joint. If you are well practised at lunges, you may wish to add dumbbells in each hand for more resistance, but make sure you don't lean forward, and keep your trunk upright.

1 set: 20, each leg. Rhythm is 2 seconds down, 2 seconds up.

Beginners – 1 set.

Advanced – 2–3 sets.

3 Press-ups

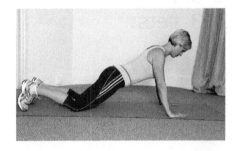
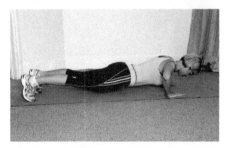

Fig.5.14

Muscles used: chest, triceps, abdominals, back.

Key points: Press-ups can be done as modified press-ups or full press-ups. Use your core (the deep abdominals and back muscles) to hold your trunk firm, and don't let your abdominals sag or let your head drop. Your hands are positioned slightly wider than your shoulders, your knees about 20 centimetres apart. Lower your chest slowly to touch the floor, then press up to full elbow extension (not locking the joints). To modify this half-press-up, bring your knees in under your hips more. To make it more difficult extend your legs and complete a full press-up.

1 set: 15. Rhythm is 2 seconds down, 2 seconds up.

Beginners – 1 set.

Advanced – 2–3 sets.

4 Hunting-dog extensions

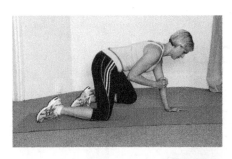

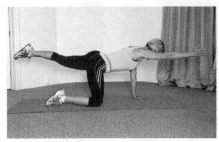

Fig.5.15

Muscles used: core stabilisers, back extensors, shoulder and butt.

Key points: Start on your hands and knees in the four-point position, spine neutral, abdominals drawn in and braced, head and neck in line with the spine, and pelvic floor zipped up. Slide the opposite hand and leg out and extend them away from the body, lifting them up to almost horizontal. Hold for 5 seconds, then slowly lower and return to the starting position. Keep your hips parallel to the floor—don't sag in the mid-region. Keep the movement slow and controlled.

1 set: Alternate 5 on each side.

Beginners – 1 set.

Advanced – 2–3 sets.

5 Tricep dips

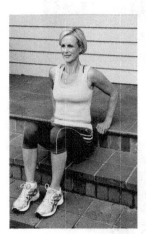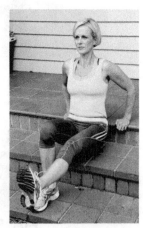

Fig.5.16

Muscles used: back of arm—triceps.

Key points: Find a step or a ledge you can put your hands on, or try flat on the floor. Align your hands under your shoulders, fingers pointing towards your toes, feet under knees, hips elevated. Bend the elbows, slowly lowering your body towards the floor, and then press through the heels of your hands and straighten them. Don't lock the elbows into full extension and keep them in close beside the body, not flaring out like chicken wings. Keep the movement continuous, bend and straighten. You can make it easier by resting your butt on the floor, or harder by lifting one foot off the floor but still keeping your hips lifted and level.

1 set: 15. Rhythm is 2 seconds down, 2 seconds up.
Beginners – 1 set.
Advanced – 2–3 sets.

6 Seated row or bent-over row with stretchy band/tube

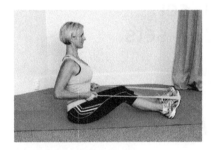

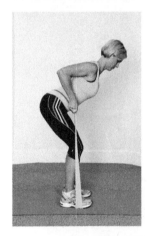

Fig.5.17

Muscles used: mid-back, biceps.
Key points: Once the band is secured around both shoes in a sitting position, or under your shoes if standing, draw in and brace your

abdominals, keeping your back firmly in the neutral spine position throughout. Pull your arms into your chest while squeezing your shoulder blades together. The bent-over row position is the more functional option, as it requires you to switch on your core muscles to stabilise your pelvis and lower back. Focus hard on maintaining good form throughout.

1 set: 15. Rhythm is 2 seconds down, 2 seconds up.

Beginners – 1 set.

Advanced – 2–3 sets.

7 Upright row

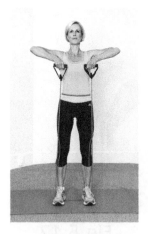

Fig.5.18

Muscles used: shoulder girdle

Key points: Secure the stretchy band under the middle of both feet, keeping your elbows out. Pull your arms up as high as your chin, maintaining a good, erect posture with a neutral spine. Lift and lower slowly.

1 set: 15 repetitions. Rhythm is 2 seconds down, 2 seconds up.

Beginners – 1 set.

Advanced – 2–3 sets.

8 Bicep curls

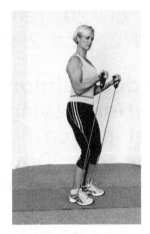

Fig.5.19

Muscles used: front of arm—biceps, forearm.

Key points: Secure the stretchy band under your feet, keeping your wrists locked in neutral position, not flexed or extended. Curl both arms up to your shoulders and slowly lower down to full extension, keeping the movement continuous.

1 set: 15 repetitions. Rhythm is 2 seconds down, 2 seconds up.

Beginners – 1 set.
Advanced – 2–3 sets.

9 Abdominals

Muscles used: abdominals, deep and superficial, plus core stabilisers.

Key points: There are exercises for each main abdominal group—transverse, obliques and rectus—plus one for the core stabiliser muscles. Perform one set of 20 repetitions for each exercise A, B, and C, and 2 static holds for D.

A Leg lowering (deep abdominals)

Starting position: Lying on your back, knees bent in, feet flat on floor.

Action—beginners: 'Draw in and brace' your abdominals (see Chapter 4 for more details). Slowly slide one of your legs from a bent position to a straight position without arching your back off the floor, and then slowly bring your leg back to the starting position. Only go as far as you can without moving your spine from the neutral position. It is better to complete the exercise with good form than to have your back arching up. As you gain strength you will be able to fully extend your leg without moving your back. Repeat 10 times on each leg.

Action—intermediates: This time your legs are elevated off the floor in a table-top position with a 90° bend at the knee. Now, maintaining your neutral back position and tightly braced abdominals, lower alternate feet so that your toes lightly touch the floor, and then lift back up again in slow, smooth controlled movements with even breathing. Right down, left down, right up, left up.

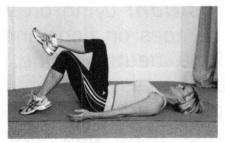

Fig.5.20

Action—advanced: From a table-top position, lower both bent legs at the same time, lightly touch toes to ground, and lift again. Make sure you are not arching your back to lift your legs up. Check by sliding your fingertips under your lower back: you should feel the same amount of pressure pressing down throughout.

B Sit-ups (superficial abdominals)

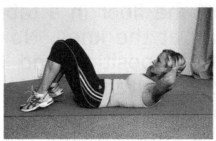

Fig.5.21

Starting position: Lying on your back with your knees bent, toes on floor and heels slightly lifted, maintain a neutral spine. Draw in and brace your abdominals, pull your belly button towards the spine, fingertips splayed loosely on the back of your head and upper neck. Your elbows should be opened out, and keep them that way throughout the exercise, chin tucked in as though you are holding a peach between it and your chest.

Action: Slowly raise your shoulders up off the floor, breathing out as you rise. Imagine a candle on your abdomen and blow it out with your exhalation as you curl up, inhale as you lower down.

1 set: 15 repetitions. Rhythm is 2 seconds up, brief pause, then 2 seconds down.

Note: Don't cup your hands together behind your head or provide any pull upwards on your neck. If you find yourself doing this, then try positioning your hands further forward on your head with your fingertips touching your temples so you can't take any weight.

C Lying crunches with a twist (obliques)

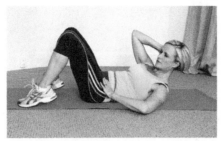

Fig.5.22

Starting position: As for sit-ups, lying with knees bent, feet flat on floor.

Action: Slowly curl up, aiming one shoulder for the opposite knee. Imagine a piece of elastic between the shoulder and your opposite hip with the two points pulling together. Slowly lower down. Exhale as you curl up, and breathe in as you lower down. You can either do 15 on one side then switch to the other, or alternate right then left.

1 set: 15 repetitions right, 15 repetitions left.

D The plank

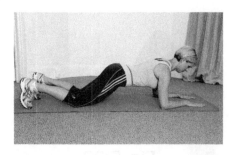

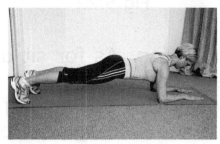

Fig.5.23

Action—beginners: Lying face down, elbows tucked under your upper body and ribcage, keeping your back in neutral. Draw in and brace your abdominals (it's the deep abdominals that stop you sagging or giving way to gravity in your middle section). Now press up so that your body is in a straight line from your knees to your forearms, lower legs on the ground, body held firm like a plank. Tuck your tailbone under and squeeze your buttock muscles. Your spine should be in line from your neck to the base of your pelvis. Now time the duration of your plank hold: start with 20 seconds and build up to 60 seconds. Keep breathing evenly throughout. Complete 2 holds.

Action—advanced: Extend your plank to your full body length by tucking your toes under and pushing up onto your feet, keeping your spine in line and body firm from head to toes. Again start with 20 seconds and build up to 60 seconds. Complete 2 holds.

10 Stretch

Complete a set of the stretches as illustrated earlier in this chapter. Congratulations, you're done! Drink a big glass of water.

Workout 2: Cross-training at home

* 30 minutes of cardiovascular training
* 30 minutes of strength training interspersed with stretching

Part 1

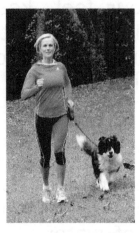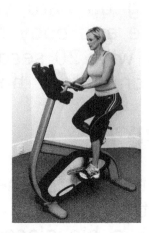

Fig.5.24

Get your walking or running shoes on and get out the door. Walk easily for the first 5 minutes, then pick up the pace, swinging your arms. Aim for an RPE (recommended perceived exertion level) of around 6–7 (out of 10): it should be 'somewhat hard' to 'hard'. If you need to increase intensity, try jogging, or interspersing jogging and walking. Vary your intensity dependent on the terrain. If it is flat you can go faster, but slow down for steep gradients. You should feel as if your heart rate and breathing rate have increased for the duration of 30 minutes, but you should not be puffing or out of breath.

If you have home cardiovascular exercise equipment (such as a bike, treadmill, etc.), you could also choose to do a 30-minute session indoors.

Stretch (Fig.5.25)

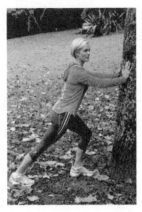 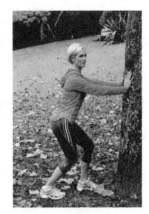

Fig.5.25

Complete Part 1 by doing both straight-knee and bent-knee calf stretches.

Part 2

As this is a cross-training workout, you will already be warmed up from doing the cardiovascular component first, so once you finish that you can launch straight into the exercises. The programme is set out in superset style, this means you partner two exercises together interspersing one set of each exercise. This will give you a time-efficient workout. For detailed descriptions and photos of each muscle targeted and action for each exercise, see the muscle-toning workout above.

With each exercise: Remember to zip up your pelvic floor muscles and brace your abdominals to provide good lower back support and strong core stabilisation throughout.

1 Squats and lunges superset (legs and butt)

1x20 squats, 15 lunges each leg, 1x20 squats, 15 lunges either leg.

Stretches x 2, alternate legs, hold for 10 seconds (Fig.5.26).

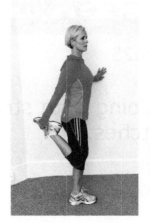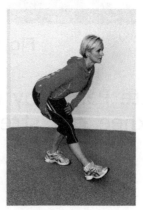

Fig.5.26

2 Press-ups and hunting-dog extensions superset (chest and back)

15 x press ups, 3 x R then 3 x L arm plus leg extensions with 5-second hold, 15 x press ups, 3 x R then 3 x L arm plus leg extensions with 5-second hold.

Stretches x 2, hold for 10 seconds.

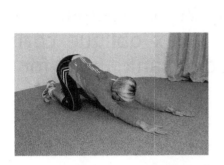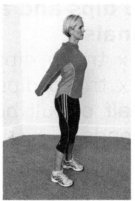

Fig.5.27

3 Bent-over row (or seated row) and upright row superset (back and shoulders)

15 x bent-over rows, 15 x upright rows, 15 x bent-over rows, 15 x upright rows.

Stretches x 2, hold for 10 seconds.

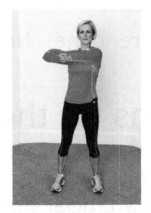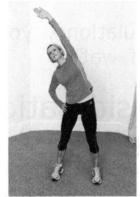

Fig.5.28

4 Tricep dips and abdominals (arms and abdominals)

15 x tricep dips, 20 x sit-ups,
15 x tricep dips, 15 x oblique curls R/L, 1 x half or full body plank, hold for 20–60 seconds.

Stretches x 2.

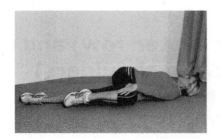 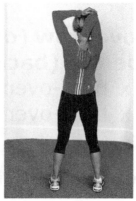

Fig.5.29

Congratulations, you're done! Now have a big drink of water.

Key considerations for the first trimester

The first trimester is a crucial time for fetal development, so whatever exercise you attempt it must always be with the knowledge and approval of your LMC (lead maternity carer).

This is not a time to take up a new high-intensity activity or anything that could put you at risk of falling or injury. However, it *is* a time to continue with the fitness programme you were participating in before conceiving. If you were a sporadic or non-existent exerciser prior to pregnancy, then it is recommended that you introduce and regularly participate in moderate exercise. Older women definitely benefit from the levels of energy felt from being more physically fit. Believe it or not, the physical energy you exert now during your pregnancy in order to get or maintain moderate fitness can enable you to be more resilient when you are a new mum.

Adjust and modify your fitness goals if you are suffering the effects of morning sickness, tiredness or any other ailment. A beginner can set a goal of gradually building up over several weeks to 20–30 minutes of exercise, three times a week at a moderate intensity. If you have regularly exercised prior to getting pregnant, then continue with your usual programme but don't overdo it: 40–60 minutes of exercise most days at a moderate intensity is plenty.

Your health and your baby's health come first; fitness comes second. But remember, unless you have a good reason to avoid it, being physically fit can enhance your pregnancy journey in many ways.

What's the ideal exercise regime?

The ideal is a combination of weight-bearing cardiovascular exercise plus strength-training sessions, which conclude with stretching after each workout.

* **Beginners** – three times a week of 30 minutes of moderate exercise
* **Experienced exercisers** – 40–60 minutes a day most days of the week, at moderate intensity.

Here is a sample programme of what you could do over a period of seven days to ensure that your programme of regular moderate exercise on most days of the week has balance and variety. It is intended as a guide only, as you need to figure out how to best incorporate regular exercise into your individual lifestyle so that it becomes an enhancement to it and not a stressor. As you know, life is never predictable and we are often faced with unforeseen demands on our time—extra work or family pressures, illness, and many other potential exercise inhibitors. Therefore a blanket prescription for exercise just doesn't work. Take the principles of balance, variety and moderation, and design your own weekly regime, one that is achievable and enjoyable for YOU. If you need help designing a programme, talk to a qualified gym instructor who should be able to give you some ideas of how to structure your workouts to achieve your goal.

Weekly guide for a currently active woman
Monday *Cardio focus.* Gym session—either a group fitness class or some sort of stationary cardiovascular machine work, 45–60 minutes' duration, RPE 5–7.

Tuesday *Strength focus.* Gym weights or pump class, 30–60 minutes.

Wednesday *Core and stretch focus.* BODYBALANCE™ class, yoga, Pilates, 30–60 minutes.

Thursday *Strength focus.* Home toning workout, strength training at gym or pump class, 45–60 minutes.

Friday *Cardio focus.* Jog, power-walk, cycle or swim, 45–60 minutes' duration, RPE 5–7.

Saturday *Combo day.* Home cross-training workout: cardio 30 minutes, toning 30 minutes (total of 60 minutes).

Sunday *Day off.* A gentle stroll or a Bare Essentials routine (see Appendix A), 15 minutes.

Key points

○ **Stop exercising** if you have any of these: injury, illness, pain or bleeding—and seek medical advice as soon as possible.

○ **Keep drinking fluids.** It is important when pregnant to maintain adequate hydration, and particularly so during the first trimester when the body's usual fluid volume levels are being adjusted. So drink before, during and after exercise. You will know you are drinking enough if your urine is pale in colour. A more potent yellow colour indicates a stronger concentration and is an indicator of potential dehydration. Keep a water-bottle handy when exercising and take frequent sips.

○ **Snacks are okay** and actually quite important to prevent dipping blood sugar levels that are often typical in the first trimester. The best sort of snack is some form of complex carbohydrate rather than a sugar-rich treat; for example, nuts, grain bread, fruit, etc. Good snack-attack packs could contain food like dried fruit and nuts, muesli bars, banana, or crackers.

○ **Rest is as important as exercise.** This is a massive time of change for your body. It needs the ability to rest, recuperate and grow a bunch of cells replicating exponentially into a baby. It also needs exercise. The key is getting the right balance so that you are not exhausted. A rule of thumb is to allow the same amount of quiet or relaxation time as you do for exercise. So if you are exercising for 30–60 minutes a day, then try to factor in about the same amount of time with your feet up (ideally).

○ **Avoid overheating.** As already discussed, pregnancy and exercise both result in the body being able to eliminate a normal build-up of heat. During the first trimester, avoid exercising in overly hot situations; for example, in the middle of a hot summer day or on holiday in a humid, hot environment. It's common sense really. Either allow your body a few days to acclimatise to a much hotter environment, or choose a time and place to exercise with a moderate temperature and adequate ventilation. Similarly, if you are suddenly at a much higher altitude then you must allow your body time to acclimatise to that, too, as oxygen availability is different from that at sea level.

○ **Above all, use your common sense.** If an activity doesn't feel good, then adjust or stop doing it.

√ Regular exercise

226

- ✓ Moderate intensity
- ✓ Hydration +
- ✓ Snacks
- ✓ Keep cool
- ✓ Rest as necessary

Chapter 6

The Second Trimester (14–27 Weeks)

Dear Diary—Eating

I wonder why I have a desire for plain food? I'm usually an olive lover, but suddenly I just want toast and butter, cheese sandwiches and bland pasta. It's weird, but I'll go with it for now. I miss creamy pâté, sushi, and sipping on a cold beer, but, as they say, 'it's not forever', and you just have to adjust your diet both for baby's sake and to respond to your changing taste buds. I have had an increased sweet tooth during this pregnancy, which can be a bit dangerous purely because my normal ability to self-check on treat foods has gone out the window proportional with my expanding belly and boobs. The other thing that is peculiar to both my pregnancies is my lack of appetite. Some days I have to psych myself up to eat. In the evening all I really crave is fruit. Speaking of cravings, as much as I'd like some I have not had any wacky ones. As yet...

Changes aplenty

Many pregnant women find this stage of their journey 'blooming lovely'. Some unlucky mums-to-be will have a few frustrating symptoms that persist, but most are now over any nausea or morning sickness, and that bone-aching tiredness also seems to lessen. In fact it is often reported that the second trimester brings a real boost of energy. Fantastic! Let's capitalise on that with keeping fit and active, but not go crazy. Even though we categorise the entire period from 14–27 weeks as the second trimester; it is worth splitting it into two further stages. The first stage is 14–20 weeks, when the hormonal inhibitors to exercise (namely nausea and tiredness) usually diminish or disappear, and the second stage of 21–27 weeks when you really become aware of your changing body shape and an increasingly protruding baby bump.

Dear Diary—Goodbye nausea
(theoretically)

I'm well into my second trimester now, well past the 12-week mark and the nausea hasn't stopped like the experts say it does. So it looks like I'm destined to put up with not just morning sickness but feeling green around the gills at any time of the day. Ripped off. I'm also bone-tired by 6pm and have had some come-home-and-just-collapse-into-bed scenarios. Everything else seems normal, but I'm just tired. I guess that's what comes from growing another human being; the body says 'time out—NOW!' I'm listening to that and not pushing on through. Actually a light dinner served in bed by one's husband is quite delightful IF you can wrangle it!

General modifications to exercising

During the first stage of the second trimester you will need to make minor modifications to your exercise regime based on the increased risk of joint laxity. This is due to the presence and ongoing effects of the hormone relaxin. You may also notice you are a little clumsier; occasionally tripping over or being a bit off-balance—this is due to your changing centre of gravity. It is probably a good idea now to lower the heel-height of the shoes you wear and to take particular care on uneven ground. The same care applies to avoiding both overheating and dehydration, particularly when exercising, as mentioned in Chapter 5.

As you progress to second stage of the second trimester, the focus is very much on continuing to do moderate exercise while not stressing your lower back and abdominal region, which will be increasingly weakened due to your abdominal muscles starting to stretch around your baby bump. You can safely assume that by about 20 weeks you will have a diastasis to some degree. Remember, the extent of the linea alba separating (the fascia between your anterior abdominals running vertically from breast bone to pelvis) varies between women and can be influenced by previous pregnancies (see Chapter 4 and Fig.4.7 for more information on diastasis). Obviously a larger diastasis means that even more care is needed when getting up and down from sitting or lying, to avoid stressing both your back and this weakened area. It is of course still important to exercise your abdominals and core muscles to maintain the corset of support they provide to your mid-region and growing baby, but the exercises will now be modified to target primarily the deep abdominals.

Regarding the baby's development during this time, it's all about *growth.* From about 14 weeks, the baby is virtually fully formed, just in miniature. It measures approximately 12cm long and has a huge head relative to the rest of its body. The placenta is providing the baby with all of its necessary oxygenated blood and nutrients.

Research shows that regular exercise over this time period improves the growth and functional capacity of the placenta, but, as already mentioned, it is important not to overdo it. You will get the most benefits for you and baby if you keep exercise to moderate levels of intensity and duration. You will know if you are overexerting yourself physically, as the placenta's function, while boosted by normal exercise, is conversely depleted by too much exercise. A well-functioning placenta results in a normal growth rate of the baby, a poorly functioning placenta results in a decreased growth rate of the baby. At your regular checks and scans, you and your LMC will quickly be able to tell if you are overdoing it by whether your baby's measurements are keeping within the normal range. If there is a drop-off in expected fetal growth rate, then you can immediately modify your exercise regime. Always err on the side of caution, especially when you are an older mum.

Another easy test to tell if any particular workout has been stressful on your baby is to monitor the baby's movements following the workout. Fetal movement varies from pregnancy to pregnancy, but in general most women will feel the baby move for the first time between 16 and 22 weeks. In the early stages it is often described as a 'quickening' or fluttering type movement. After about 28 weeks it is definitely more of a 'kick'. Some babies are more active than others. Fetal activity is affected by sleep, sound, time of day, and the mother's activity level. Typically, exercising moderately will increase the baby's movements following the session. On average your baby should move at least two or three times in the 30 minutes following exercise, but remember that this is an average only. If you are concerned about a decrease or absence of your baby's movements, contact your LMC. It will help if you keep a note of when you last felt any movement and of any subsequent moves until you see your LMC. It may be nothing more than your baby taking a rest, but it is always worth a check if you have any concerns.

Dear Diary—Where are you, waist?

Where has my waist gone? The reality is that it is LONG gone. It's like someone has grabbed a spatula and filled in the contour that used to be my waist. I miss you, waist, as you meant I could put my hands on my hips and strike a pose; now I'm grabbing my bilateral muffin tops. Yesterday at work I was sitting at my desk and I suddenly felt tired. Not just ebbing tired, but more a sense of having any energy sucked out of me with a vacuum. I got home and tumbled into bed. I was meant to go along to a cycle class this morning, but I cancelled that in favour of a walk with the dog. I think there are some weeks when you feel more on top of things than others, and clearly this is a low-energy week. I need to maintain my energy levels, so I am adapting my exercise plan. There's got to be a benefit or two in being an older mum (relatively speaking) and I'd like to think it's wisdom!

Exercise and side-effects

Placenta praevia

The placenta usually sits high in the uterus, either on the front or back wall. However, if it is lying over part of the cervix or over the entire cervix, it is called 'placenta praevia'. This is a major problem in late pregnancy and labour, as the baby cannot advance down the birth canal through the placenta. The sooner the situation is detected the better, as careful monitoring is necessary, and most likely a caesarean section will be planned to avoid risks to the baby and the mother. It may be evident at a 20-week scan, but if it is detected at that stage your LMC will advise you on appropriate modified exercise or rest. The majority of placenta praevia detected at the 20-week scan actually resolve themselves due to the rapid growth of the uterus in late pregnancy. Often the first sign of a praevia occurring is recurrent light bleeding. If that occurs, *stop* any exercising and do not resume until you have seen and discussed the situation with your LMC.

Anaemia (iron deficiency)

This is quite common during pregnancy due to the change in blood volume, and it is often picked up during routine pregnancy blood tests. If you are found to be low on iron, your LMC will recommend a suitable supplement, plus you can also eat iron-rich foods. (See Chapter 2.) If you are anaemic, the sorts of symptoms you may experience are fatigue, shortness of breath, paleness and low blood pressure. If you have any of these signs, then it is worth getting your iron levels checked. Once you have built your body stores back up you should be able to continue exercising. For the period in which you are increasing your iron intake, decrease your exercise intensity and duration.

Pre-term labour

It is advisable to seek advice from your LMC even if you are just getting cramping in response to exercise. Towards the end of the second trimester and increasingly in the third, some women will get sporadic uterine cramps when exercising. If the cramps stop shortly after exercising there is generally no problem, but if they persist for 20–30 minutes or more, then true labour may not be far away. Seek expert advice from your LMC as soon as possible. Pre-term labour is defined as any series of contractions that occur before 37 weeks' gestation.

Hypertension and pre-eclampsia (toxaemia)

Hypertension means high blood pressure. Mildly elevated high blood pressure during pregnancy often resolves with rest. High blood pressure combined with swelling of the hands, feet and face often signals a condition called pre-eclampsia. The cause of this condition is not fully known, but it is believed to be brought on by a combination of genes, immune system and environmental factors. Pre-eclampsia affects the placenta, reducing blood supply to both the baby and the mother. You will need to be carefully monitored by your LMC if you have either high blood pressure or preeclampsia, and exercise is *not* recommended.

Gestational diabetes

This condition is likely to be temporary and usually disappears after birth. It affects 1–3% of women, and its onset is most typically during the second trimester. Maternal age is an established risk factor for gestational diabetes mellitus (GDM). Any woman over the age of 25 should be routinely tested for it, as the risk of GDM increases significantly and progressively from this age onwards. If you are in the 35+ age group you have a statistically higher risk of developing GDM.

It is caused by the pregnancy hormones affecting the insulin levels in some women. Insulin is normally produced by the pancreas, and is used by the body to remove sugar from the blood and make it available to the cells for energy. Without enough insulin, sugar levels in the blood rise, making the person feel unwell. A blood test to detect sugar levels is usually carried around 26 weeks, although it may be picked up in other routine testing before then.

If you have gestational diabetes it will be monitored throughout pregnancy, but usually regular moderate exercise is recommended. In fact, exercise plays quite an important role, as it can increase the efficiency or potency of your body's own insulin, allowing you to maintain a more normal range of blood sugar and possibly even resulting in you having to use less insulin. Cardiovascular exercise and strength training are both beneficial. Exercise in general also helps control appetite and will help with keeping your weight gain within acceptable norms. Your LMC is also likely to suggest changes to your diet.

Symphysis pubis dysfunction

The pubic symphysis is a joint at the front of your pelvis. The two pelvic bones are held together by a strong fibrous joint that outside of pregnancy moves very little. However, during pregnancy, as with other ligaments and tendons in your body, this joint will become increasingly lax due to the hormone relaxin. Any strain or jerk to the area may strain and inflame the area. Pubic symphysis problems can take a long time to heal and are very painful, so from the second trimester on reduce your risk by avoiding movements where you are separating your legs, like getting in and out of the car, climbing over a gate, etc. Exercises that maintain good strength in your buttocks are also helpful in maintaining pelvic stability. In particular, the gluteus medius on the outside of the hip should be strengthened; side leg lifts and standing balance work are good for this. Please be careful to not overstretch the hip area; for example, with yoga. You need to maintain hip strength and stability, not laxity. Remember, pregnancy hormones are acting to relax the ligaments around your joints, so don't exacerbate this.

Dear Diary—Burping and snoring

I'm totally over burping. Completely! At any time of the day I seem to be getting mild indigestion which results in me burping. Uggggh. At least it's not vomiting, I suppose. Be thankful for small things. I've tried antacids but they don't seem to have much effect, so I guess I'm just destined to be windy. I really hope it stops once I've given birth!

Hubby tells me I snore. I would like to formally state this is **not usual.** It's evidently quite common with pregnant women, and increasingly so as the pregnancy progresses, but that fact doesn't make it any less annoying for the bed partner. He's too scared to wake me up or roll me over when I start honking, as during this trimester I'm lucky if I get a good sleep at the best of times. So the audible inconvenience for him is overridden by wanting a refreshed and rested wife. Poor hubby! Now he knows how I feel when HE snores, which is frequently and he doesn't have pregnancy as an excuse.

Care and posture

Getting up and down

As your baby bump gets more pronounced, you should avoid the old heave-ho manoeuvre when getting up out of a chair, up from lying, or in and out of a car. This only puts extra strain and stress on your already stretched and weakened abdominal area, especially as the diastasis (gap) appears on the front abdominal wall. Roll or shift to the side, get your legs underneath you, and use your strong leg muscles to propel yourself up and your arms to assist. Avoid movements that result in the abdominal region doming or bulging out forwards.

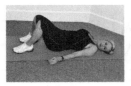 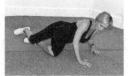 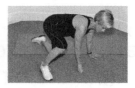

Fig.6.1

Similarly, take extra care with any lifting. Think first; plan your lift. Squat down, draw in and brace your abdominals, pull the load close to your body and keep it there. Bend your knees and power up using your large leg muscles to take the load. *Never* twist and lift. If you want to change direction, move your feet, not your back.

Lying on your back

For many years, pregnant women have been advised to avoid lying on their backs from the second trimester. This conservative advice is based on a potential problem that may occur with some women. From about 16 weeks when you are lying face up, the size and weight of your uterus can press down on a major blood vessel (the vena cava), restricting blood flow and lowering blood pressure for both mum and baby. This results in symptoms like dizziness, shortness of breath, or even, in extreme cases, fainting. They have even given the condition a name: maternal supine hypotension syndrome. Remember that this is cautionary advice, so whenever possible avoid being on your back for any longer than a few minutes at a time, but don't panic about rolling over on to your back or moving through the position when you are exercising.

Standing for long periods

Another piece of cautionary advice—to avoid standing for long periods—is to prevent potential circulation problems, like the swelling of the lower limbs and feet, as well as a sore back due to your altered size and shape. It really only applies to those pregnant women who stand still for long periods of time. This may be the case at your workplace when you have to stand stationary behind a shop counter or similar. Easy remedies are to do some foot pedalling while standing, lift your heels and change your weight from side to side, or consider asking your employer for a suitable chair that gives you good back support, thus intersperse standing with periods of sitting. Practise some standing pelvic tilts (tucking your tailbone under) to ease your lower back. Take any opportunity to walk a little, as movement is better for your back and legs than standing still.

Cardiovascular exercise

A reminder

If you experience any of these symptoms during exercise, simply stop the activity and discuss it with your LMC:

* excessive shortness of breath
* headache or dizziness
* pain—in particular chest or abdomen pain
* nausea or vomiting
* light vaginal bleeding—stop and have it evaluated
* contractions
* deep back or pubic pain
* cramping in the lower abdomen
* sudden swelling of hands, face and ankles
* unusual change in the baby's movements—usually a marked decrease
* amniotic fluid leakage.

If you have had to cease exercising during your first trimester due to pregnancy complications but have now been given the all-clear by your LMC, then treat yourself as a beginner for the first few weeks that you resume activity. Do a few easy-level workouts first and let your body adapt. Depending on how long you have had to cease any exercise, be aware that you may not get back to your pre-pregnancy exercise level, but that's okay.

So long as you are exercising moderately, you and your baby will get the health benefits.

Exercise tips for the second trimester

Pay particular attention to allowing adequate time to warm up and cool down, at least 5–10 minutes for each. Keep your exercise intensity now to around 5–6 RPE (rate of perceived exertion; see Chapter 1). Dress in layers to avoid overheating, make sure you have water readily available and take frequent sips to avoid dehydration. Your external shape is now changing to show your belly protruding, so you may get increased lower back tension or twinges in your hips and pelvis. Use a low-grade draw-in and abdominal bracing action to provide support for your lower back and tummy. Check your upright posture when exercising, to avoid over-arching your lower back. You may find that you naturally adopt a wider stance in standing to provide a more stable base of support. Pelvic tilts are a good exercise to do when you are standing still, at the kitchen sink, talking on the phone, etc.

Suitable second-trimester cardiovascular exercise

✓ **Walking** Remind yourself about good upright posture while you are walking, brace your lower abdominals, and avoid arching your lower back. Think about drawing your hip bones together, your abdominals in, and zip up those pelvic floor muscles. Keep your shoulders pressed down and back. Remember the 'talk test': you should be able to maintain a reasonable conversation while walking, but probably not be able to sing the national anthem! Make sure you have a sturdy, supportive pair of walking shoes, and take particular care negotiating rough ground or cracked pavements. Your balance and equilibrium will continue to change as your pregnancy progresses. When negotiating high steps (for example, climbing over gates or fences), keep your legs together as much as possible to prevent straining your pubic symphysis—the fibrous joint at the front of your pelvis. Pregnancy hormones make this increasingly unstable, and the action of lifting your one leg up and out could give it a nasty twinge. Prevention with the pubic symphysis joint is far better than cure. During the second trimester, beginners should aim to build up to 30 minutes' walking duration three times a week; those more active can aim for 60 minutes most days of the week. Walking is a great low-impact exercise option to slot in several times a week, alternating with your other fitness activities, providing you have no pelvic instability issues. As your pregnancy progresses you might find that it takes more effort to do exactly the same walking route that you did during the first trimester—this is normal.

✓ **Running/Jogging** If you have already been running or jogging regularly throughout your first trimester, you can continue on, but be aware of your changing centre of gravity and decreasing ability to balance. Towards the second half of this trimester, as you physically expand more and your ligaments and tendons continue to soften due to the presence of the pregnancy hormone relaxin, you may find it uncomfortable to run downhill or run at all. The total duration of your run/jog may also need to be decreased. Listen to your body, note your levels of tiredness and keep your LMC fully informed of your exercise programme. Some days you will feel like moving a bit faster, others you won't. On those slower days, do a fast power-walk instead, so you are pulling back on the intensity but still reaping the benefits of getting out in the fresh air. Choose your terrain carefully and take particular care to avoid uneven ground. If your route does involve a steep downhill slope or steps, then slow down to a walk while keeping your knees soft to cushion your foot strike impact. Increase your warm-up and cool-down durations, allowing at least 5–10 minutes for each. Gradually increase your pace, begin with a walking warm-up, then progress to an easy jog and then to running. Taper off as you complete your run in the same manner. Be careful with running uphill as your heart rate will elevate quickly. Consider a workout with a run/walk combination, where you jog on the flat and walk up or down steep hills. Take water with you to keep hydrated, and dress appropriately so you can peel off a layer as your body heat increases.

√ **Outdoor cycling** If you have not cycled before becoming pregnant, it is probably not the best choice of exercise at this stage; exercise on a stationary cycle instead. If you are already proficient on a bike, then just be aware of not putting yourself in a situation where you might take a tumble or fall. It is a potentially riskier way of exercising than other modes, but the choice is yours. Now is not the time to take up mountain-bike riding!

Home-based and gym cardio equipment

A workout that utilises several different pieces of cardio equipment is a good option for achieving moderate fitness while combating any boredom that often accompanies using indoor machines like steppers or treadmills. Try a warm-up of 5–10 minutes then 10–15 minutes on two or three different machines with short change-over times in between.

√ **Stationary bike** Avoid pelvic strain when getting on or off the bike by sitting your butt on the seat from the side and swivelling your legs around. Don't hike your leg up too high (see the pubic symphysis advice earlier). Towards stage two of the second trimester, you may find your tummy starting to get in the way of your legs when you are leaning forward, so choose a bike that allows you to adjust both seat height and handlebar height to allow you to achieve a more upright sitting posture. When setting your seat, put it at a height that allows about a 10° bend in your knee at the base of the pedal circle. If your seat height is too high, you will end up dropping your pelvis to either side as your leg straightens, and that can be problematic for your back. Intersperse periods of leaning forward to the handle bars with sitting upright to ease any strain on your lower back, and while sitting upright do some backward shoulder rolls. From the second trimester some women find a recumbent bike a good option, or, if your baby bump is getting in the way of your legs, then opt for the treadmill.

> *I found during my second trimester that a resistance level of zero (i.e., no resistance added) on the elliptical trainer still elevated my heart rate sufficiently to provide a good moderate cardiovascular workout.*

√ **Elliptical trainer** This machine requires reasonable balance, but its motion is low-impact so it's a good choice for this trimester. It also uses arms and leg movements together (if you are on a machine that has moveable arms), so this will raise your heart rate more quickly than some other cardio machine options. When warming up, just do the leg movements, then add in the arm activity later. Just be aware of keeping your RPE (rate of perceived exertion level) to around 5–6, so when exercising you would describe your intensity or effort as 'somewhat hard'.

√ **Stepper** From the second trimester it is important to maintain pelvic alignment to avoid stress and strain on your lower back and pelvis, and the action of changing your weight from one step to the other could prove troublesome. Make sure you maintain a good upright posture, do a low-grade abdominal brace throughout, and zip up your pelvic floor muscles. Also don't have the stepping range too high; a mid-sized movement is preferable to a movement that replicates high knee-lifting. Avoid the stepper if you have sacroiliac pain, as it will only exacerbate it.

√ **Rower** Correct technique is vital to get benefit from this low-impact upper- and lower-body exercise. If you are unsure on the action, then ask an instructor to show you the correct set-up and movement. You may find rowing fine for the first half of this trimester, but once your tummy begins to touch your knees when performing the movement it is time to choose another activity. Switch on your core abdominal muscles and draw your belly button towards your spine to give extra support to your lower back.

√ **Treadmill** A good piece of equipment for beginners as it is adaptable to all fitness levels by adjusting both intensity and gradient. You can walk or jog or do a combination of the two, depending on how you are feeling on the day. The same sort of considerations apply as listed for walking and jogging, above, but of course on this machine you don't have to worry about uneven ground—just pay attention so you don't daydream and fall off!

Water-supported exercise

In water, you will feel a sense of weightlessness that is often a welcome relief, especially for the latter half of pregnancy. The buoyancy of water takes the pressure off sore backs and other joints, and is a great medium in which to relax and just enjoy the sensation of floating when you have finished exercising. Providing you are in water with a temperature of 27–30° Celsius, you should be able to avoid overheating. Don't jump or dive in, especially after 20 weeks' pregnancy, as both actions provide potential risk to you and your baby. It is always a good idea to shower off after a pool workout to wash off any chlorine or other pool chemicals.

√ **Swimming** Swimming is an excellent activity to continue with or take up during your second trimester, especially if you are finding other forms of impact exercise (such as jogging or classes) uncomfortable. If you are having any discomfort or pain with your pubic symphysis joint at the front of the pelvis, the breaststroke action with the legs may further exacerbate it, so avoid that movement. Try normal freestyle or backstroke, which keep the legs closer together. Butterfly is one stroke to avoid from this stage on, as the action may provide too much arch through your lower back. (But full credit to you for being able to do butterfly in the first place!) Remember, swimming is not a weight-bearing exercise, and research shows that weight-bearing exercise is important for preventing osteoporosis (brittle bone disease). So a balanced programme would include swimming exercise plus some walking or weight-bearing aerobic exercise each week.

√ **Aqua jogging** You can either do this in chest- to shoulder-depth water and just jog along the pool floor using your arms and legs, or you can do it in deep water with the use of a floatation device. The floatation vest (often hired on-site) straps firmly around your trunk, helping to keep you in the upright position. Pump your arms up and down as if you were running, and keep your fingers together. Try experimenting with flat-blade hand positions to get more or less resistance from the water as you jog along. Lifting your knees higher creates a bigger movement and more water resistance, and will elevate your heart rate. Even when jogging along at a decent speed and with a good range of movement, you still should be able to conduct a conversation. Beginners can start with a 5–10 minute session and build up from there. If you are a regular exerciser, then aim for 30 minutes and consider tagging on some swimming lengths. Aqua jogging can be a bit boring if you are doing it by yourself, so invite someone to join you in the pool, perhaps someone at a similar stage of pregnancy. Consider, too, alternating between swimming and aqua jogging.

√ **Aqua aerobics** Again, as the water is supporting your body these sorts of exercise classes are brilliant for the second and even third trimesters. Make sure the instructor is aware that you are pregnant, and modify the moves accordingly. Some facilities may even run specific pregnancy aqua aerobics. Most classes will involve using the water to provide resistance to your movements, and have the usual class structure of warm-up, exercise session and then cool-down and stretching. Don't overdo it; watch for feeling dizzy or light-headed, and if you experience these symptoms get to the edge of the pool and take a break or end your workout. If you have any pubic symphysis pain, then side squatting moves used to move down the pool may be aggravating, so when everyone is travelling sideways just turn fronton and walk in the same direction.

Group fitness classes

Group fitness classes create an environment that is typically encouraging and upbeat, which provides good motivation to exercise. They are also timetabled, which means you are more likely to attend as you have made an appointment to exercise at a specific time. If you have not been a regular class participant until now, I would caution you against beginning any class unless it is tailored for pregnant women or offers clear movement modifications. It is not the time to take up high-impact aerobics, step, boxing or similar. Pregnant beginner exercisers who are in the second trimester are far better taking up walking, swimming or using stationary cardio machines to get low-risk but effective aerobic exercise. However, if you have regularly attended classes, then the second trimester will involve some modification to your routines.

In this section I outline pregnancy modifications for a variety of Les Mills classes as their group fitness programme is available in 80 countries worldwide, but of course they are not the only class options. There are many other suitable exercise classes you can attend at gyms and in the local community. If the class you choose to attend is similar in content to those outlined here then cast your eye over the modifications and adapt as necessary. As a general rule, for any class you should always let the instructor know you are pregnant so they can provide additional cueing and offer alternative movements that are more suitable for pregnancy. If you feel the instructor does not have the knowledge to modify the movements accordingly, then use your own sensible judgement and always err on the side of caution. Do less rather than more.

√ **Cycle classes** These classes are often viewed as an intense exercise option, but they don't need to be, as you can adjust the resistance on the pedals to get whatever workout level you choose. Just make sure that during your second trimester you don't get swept up by the music and instructor and end up pushing yourself too hard. Using a heart-rate monitor during the class is a great idea to give you immediate feedback on your intensity level. Also perhaps choose a bike at the rear of the class so you don't feel self-conscious when modifying the moves or slowing down compared with the rest of the class. Your RPE (rate of perceived exertion) should be around 5–6, described as 'somewhat hard'; one notch down from what you attempted in the first trimester. If you are a beginner, ask for plenty of advice on setting up the bike correctly for your height and size, as most are extremely adjustable. Do a beginners' class or an introduction class to see if it is to your liking. Most bike pedals also have two options for footwear, cleats for cycle shoes on one side and on the other an adjustable toe-basket that fits any gym shoe.

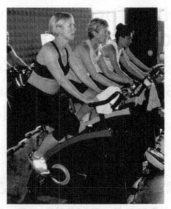

Fig.6.2

Towards the second half of this trimester, as your belly starts to protrude forward more, lift your handlebars higher so you are not leaning as far forward. Make sure you choose a bike located where there is good ventilation, and have water to sip throughout the session. Good cycling technique applies even more during pregnancy, where you want to avoid straining your pelvis. Try to maintain a good midline position and avoid lateral pelvic tilt down on each side.

From the middle of the second trimester (about 20 weeks) avoid standing out of the saddle for any length of time, as this will raise your heart rate too high and further risk pelvic instability. Your lower abdominals should be contracted to support your lower back. Remind yourself to pull up your pelvic floor muscles, and use your time in the class to do several sets of pelvic floor exercises. You may like to use a gel seat cover for extra padding. Wear appropriate layers of clothing so you do not overheat. Stretch your arms back and roll your shoulders back regularly to maintain good erect upper body posture. Don't feel any pressure to keep up with everything the class is asked to do. You are pregnant, not competing in the Tour de France! It's probably advisable not to cycle on consecutive days, but alternate classes with something else like walking or swimming.

√ **Aerobic classes** By the second trimester you should start limiting the high-impact moves and replacing them with the low-impact versions. Most instructors will give you options of intensity. You may also wish to switch to a low-impact class (like BODYVIVE™, a Les Mills group fitness class). Turns or twists are also reasonably risky, due to your changing centre of balance and increasingly lax ligaments due to pregnancy hormones, so avoid complex or twisting moves. Avoid sit-ups in abdominal tracks.

√ **Step classes** Modify the intensity of your activity during this sort of class. Work within a RPE of 5–6 and opt for all the low-impact moves. For step classes, if you have been using two levels under the step, drop down to one or use just the top platform itself. Avoid twisting movements, and if there is a sequence of exercise using this type of action, then just march or low jog on the spot until you can join in again. Sip water frequently.

√ **Kick-boxing/Cross-fit type classes** These are not recommended during pregnancy, and cease mixed martial arts-type classes from the second trimester onwards.

√ **Circuit classes** This type of class can have bursts of very intense activity, interspersed with more static exercising. Because of that structure, you may feel that the amount of modifying you need to do makes a circuit class generally a poor choice from the second trimester onwards. If you do wish to participate, then avoid: any activity that may result in a fall or hard contact with someone else in the class; lying on your tummy; sit-ups; twisting and high-impact propulsion moves. Moderate your heart rate to no higher than 140–160bpm maximum.

✓ **BODYBALANCE™** The theme of this Les Mills trademarked programme is suitable for pregnancy: gentle, low-impact exercise involving breathing, stretching and strengthening. With some modifications it is a suitable choice for this trimester and beyond. Gyms offering BODYBALANCE™ classes should be able to provide you with a specific pregnancy guide for this class that includes photos of the recommended modifications for pregnant participants. If you are new to this class, make sure you advise the instructor you are pregnant so they can provide verbal cues for appropriate track modifications, and if possible get them to demonstrate to you the alternative recommended moves. It is best to do this prior to attending a class. Even though it is a stretch-and-flex type of class, it can be performed intensely if you push every move to its limit. It is advisable while you are pregnant to pull back from maximum participation and to just attempt moves with moderate intensity and range. Don't feel you need to keep up with the instructor or the rest of the class.

General BODYBALANCE™ modifications

Have your feet slightly wider than hip-distance apart to give you a stronger base of support. Instead of jumping your feet apart, step one out at a time to avoid stressing your pelvic joints and pelvic floor muscles. When stretching forward from standing or sitting, keep your legs apart to give your baby bump plenty of room. Only stretch to within your usual range of motion, don't push further and overstretch. Avoid positions called 'three-legged dog' and 'standing split'. Modify your routine to do what feels comfortable for you. Ensure good upright posture in standing, don't do any leaning back beyond neutral, and tuck your tailbone under to achieve good pelvic alignment, especially with movements like lunges. Modify any repetitive stepping lunge move into a static lunge or squat position. Work at your own pace and take a break whenever you need to; you don't need to do every move or every track. Comfortable positions to rest in are 'child's pose' or 'seated star pose'. Each class follows a predictable format, so here are more detailed modifications for the sort of moves you will encounter in each specific track.

Specific track modifications

• **Track 2—sun salutations** Yoga basis. Feet wider than hip-width apart, taking particular care when moving quickly from standing to lunging. Replace 'crocodile', 'cobra' and 'up dog' poses with 'cat stretch', if desired.

• **Track 4—balance** Your centre of gravity is changing as your shape alters, so balancing is more difficult. Modify balance poses from one to both feet on the ground if necessary, or use the wall for support.

• **Track 6—core abdominals** After 16 weeks, avoid lying on your back for any length of time (i.e., longer than a few minutes). If you experience dizziness lying on your back, roll to the side and sit up, and change to doing deep abdominal tightening on your hands and knees instead. If you are comfortable on your back, do those deep abdominal exercises which strengthen the core, remembering to draw in and brace the abdominals, but eliminate any curl-up or twisting type move. A good abdominal exercise modification for this trimester is lying on your back with bent knees and performing alternate single leg raises. The instructor may demonstrate some alternative moves suitable for you, like 'bridging' or a 'hindi squat'; take care with the latter move if you have any pelvic or pubic symphysis pain.

• **Track 7—core back** Avoid lying on your stomach for obvious reasons, and replace with four-point kneeling. Use the 'camel' pose instead of the 'bow' pose. Keep your legs strong, your chest lifted, and head and neck relaxed.

● **Track 8—twists** When twisting, turn away from the bent knee and minimise the turn movement so that there is no compression of your baby.

● **Track 9—forward bends** Legs apart when bending forward, and avoid compression of your baby bump. If you experience any dizziness when your head is down, come up to a back flat position with bent knees, and support your body weight with your elbows resting on your thighs.

● **Track 10—relaxation/meditation** Lie on your side rather than your back, especially towards the end of the second trimester.

The information for pregnancy modifications for Les Mills BODYBALANCE™ has been supplied by Les Mills International and specifically addresses pregnancy modifications recommended for this class (as at 2012).

Dear Diary—Bedtime with Mr Blue

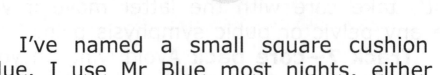

I've named a small square cushion Mr Blue. I use Mr Blue most nights, either on one side or the other as a pillow under my top knee. This is supposed to reduce the drag downwards on your pelvic joints, which by now are getting soft and flexible, and supposedly a whole night in an errant position might leave me with back ache. Anyway, I have duly bonded with Mr Blue. I notice that if I lie on my left side the baby kicks moderately, but if I like on my right I get a decent pummelling. Baby is particularly active between 8 and 10pm at night, or maybe that's just when I slow down and am more aware of the movements. It's not flutters either, as some books describe it, it's full-on soccer kicks followed by what feels like a 360° body roll. The past week has been less than ideal, with baby also having a good kick at about 2am! I'm not ready yet for broken sleep—there will be plenty of that once the little acrobat has ejected from the womb.

Strength training

BODYPUMP™

If you were doing a Les Mills BODYPUMP™ class before becoming pregnant or throughout your first trimester, then you can continue on, but with certain exercise modifications. It is not the time to start this class if you are an absolute beginner with strength training. Advise the instructor that you are pregnant so that they can specifically cue appropriately modified moves. Gyms providing the Les Mills range of group fitness classes should be able to provide you with a BODYPUMP™ pregnancy guide.

General BODYPUMP™ modifications

Keep a slightly wider stance than normal to provide a more stable base. Pregnancy is not a time to increase your weights, and as your pregnancy progresses, reduce your workload in the tracks by lowering your weights. Work at your own pace and within a shorter range of movement as your pregnancy progresses. No jerking or jarring. Don't work to failure in any track. Maintain good core muscle activation, and be aware of good erect posture in standing with a neutral spine. Avoid leaning back or overarching your lower back. Incline the bench for floor tracks. Take care getting down on to the bench, and move out of lying on the bench by rolling to the side, not sitting forwards. You will need to modify the usual abdominal exercises to focus on deep abdominals or obliques, or skip the abdominal track completely and do some gentle stretching. For the first part of the second trimester you may find lying on your back presents no problem, but from about 16 weeks on it is best to adapt the abdominal exercises into side lying or up on hands and knees. If you experience any dizziness or nausea (symptoms of supine hypotensive syndrome), move out of the lying position by rolling to the side and then sit up. Avoid holding your breath, as this can elevate your blood pressure. Remember to exhale as you exert effort, and keep breathing evenly throughout.

Specific track modifications

● **Track 2—legs/squats** Squat position should be slightly wider, with feet wider than shoulder-distance apart. Avoid excessive curvature in your lower back, engage your lower abdominals and draw them in. Zip up your pelvic floor. Breathe evenly throughout the exercise. Decrease the load.

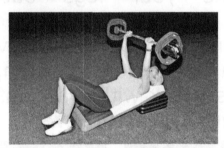

Fig.6.3

● **Track 3—chest** Incline the bench for comfort. Take care getting on and off, rolling to the side rather than sitting forward and up.
● **Track 4—back/gluteals/hamstrings** Maintain a wider than normal stance, and consider using plates rather than the bar for clean-and-press moves. Keep your wrists strong and slightly extended during the clean phase of the clean-and-press action. Focus on rolling

the shoulders back and squeezing your shoulder blades together; this helps maintain strength in your upper back as more load is placed on your posture through increasing breast size. If you feel dizzy or light-headed when doing the press above your head move, modify and use an upright row instead.

● **Track 5—arms/triceps** Incline the bench for extensions, presses and pullovers. If you prefer to not lie down, then try a seated position for tricep extension work and use a plate instead of the bar; intersperse this with tricep kickbacks on hands and knees. Dips off the edge of the bench are fine, but you may need to take your legs out further to accommodate your baby bump. For any of the exercise options with weights above your head, don't feel an obligation to complete all the repetitions, just work within a comfortable range and remember to breathe evenly.

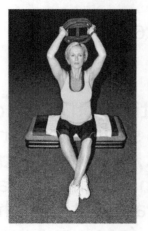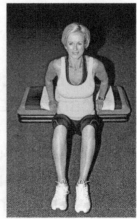

Fig.6.4

● **Track 6—legs/lunges** If you have any history of sacroiliac problems or pelvic instability, use a squat instead of a lunge. For the first stage of the second trimester you may wish to continue with lunges, but don't bother using any weights. Avoid stepping lunges; just stick with the static lunge or choose a squat option instead. Pay attention to correct body posture by really focusing on keeping your trunk upright without leaning back. Engage and pull in your lower abdominals throughout the exercise to support your lower back.

● **Track 7—abdominals** For the first stage of the second trimester you may wish to continue lying on your back, but switch any sit-up move for pelvic tilts or heel drops which targets your deep abdominals. Another option is to do abdominal bracing in four-point kneeling.

The information for pregnancy modifications for Les Mills BODYPUMP™ has been supplied by Les Mills International and specifically addresses pregnancy modifications recommended for this class (as at 2012).

Own strength-training programme

If you have been participating in resistance training with weights or machines at a gym, then for the first stage of the second trimester

(12–20 weeks) decrease your weights by about 5–10%. As you progress into the second stage of the second trimester (20–28 weeks), decrease your weights a further 5–10%. You should be able to complete 10–15 repetitions of each exercise comfortably, with two or three sets. Never exercise to a level where you feel you are straining hard or 'working to failure'. As has already been mentioned, this is not a time to increase your weights; it is a maintenance phrase with a gradual reduction in the loads you are lifting.

If you are considering introducing strength training in your second trimester, then I would highly recommend you enlisting the services of a qualified personal trainer who can give you a suitable programme. Make sure the personal trainer has specific experience with exercise prescription for pregnant women. In general, you will be performing high repetitions (10–20) with one to three sets per exercise. A circuit style combination of exercises works well.

Machine or free-weights strength exercises for the second trimester (with modifications)

If you are unsure of technique, get a gym instructor to demonstrate the correct action throughout the exercise.

LOWER BODY

1 Leg-press

Seated or inclined, limit the range of movement so that your knees avoid compressing your baby bump. Don't simply flare out your knees—this can put extra strain on the pelvis.

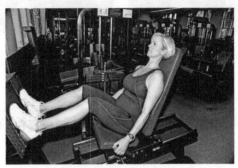

Fig.6.5

2 Squats with barbell in front of your body

See the squat technique photo for correct form. Switch to dumbbells if using a barbell in front proves too difficult to manage.

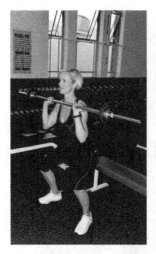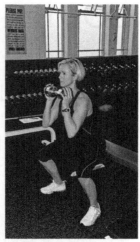

Fig.6.6

3 Seated leg extension and seated hamstring curl

Sit with your back supported, and switch on your deep abdominals to brace as you either extend your lower legs up or pull your heels down and back.

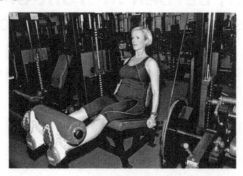

Fig.6.7

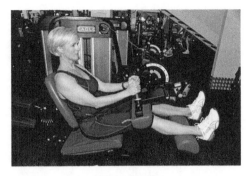

Fig.6.8

UPPER BODY

1 Lat pull-down

Ensure good sitting posture, then bring the bar down in front of your body.

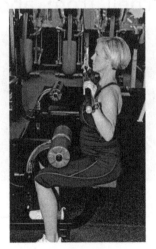

Fig.6.9

2 Seated row

Maintain a sitting position with a neutral spine and shoulders down, then focus on squeezing the shoulder blades together.

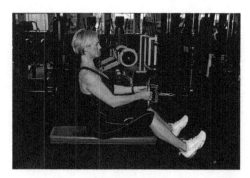

Fig.6.10

3 Bent-over row

Maintain a straight back and tilt from the hips. This is a very good exercise for core stability of the mid-region, and can be done in a standing or seated position. Try dumbbells rather than a barbell from about 20 weeks.

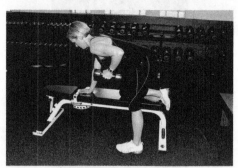

Fig.6.11

4 Chest-press on an incline bench

As your second trimester progresses you can increase the pitch of the incline to bring you more upright. From the second stage of this trimester, use dumbbells rather than a barbell. Maintain your spine pressed down into the bench. Avoid splitting your legs wide apart; consider using a step or a bench to put your feet on so you can keep your knees no wider than hip-distance apart. A similar incline bench position can be used for other free-weights exercises like flys and bicep curls.

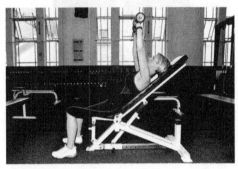

Fig.6.12

ARMS

1 Tricep press-down

As your baby bump grows, you may find that it becomes difficult to fully extend the bar, in which case do single-arm press-downs or switch to tricep kickbacks.

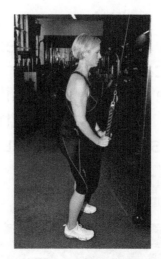

Fig.6.13

2 Bicep curl

These can be done standing or sitting. If your baby bump begins to impede the barbell movement, then switch to dumbbells.

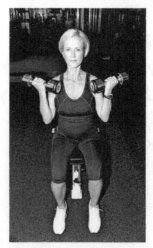

Fig.6.14

3 Lateral raise

Standing or sitting, drop your shoulders down before you start, then begin the movement.

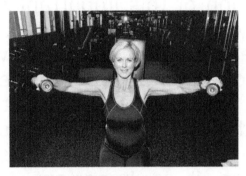

Fig.6.15

4 Upright row

Do this with a bar or dumbbells.

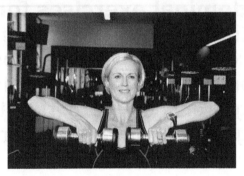

Fig.6.16

ABDOMINALS

Supine hypotensive syndrome results in dizziness, nausea, etc. It is caused by the weight of the growing baby and the uterus

274

pushing down and obstructing the major blood vessel returning blood to the heart from the lower part of the body—the inferior vena cava. Any obstruction of this important blood vessel can make you feel light-headed, dizzy, and even cause fainting. Not all women get symptoms of supine hypotensive syndrome when lying on their backs, but it is prudent to restrict the amount of time you spend in this position after about 16 weeks' gestation. At this stage it is important to focus on strengthening the deep abdominals, so sit-ups are off the menu, and the length of time you hold a static contraction should also decrease.

Suitable abdominal exercises for this stage

Drawing in and bracing abdominals while on all fours—targeting the deep abdominals. (See Chapter 4 for exercise progressions.)

Side lying crunches—targeting the obliques.

Side lying plank with knees bent and elbow support.

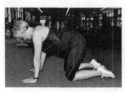 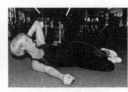 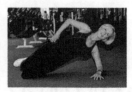

Fig.6.16

Flexibility

By the second trimester you may become aware of the effects of the pregnancy hormone relaxin which acts on tendons and ligaments throughout your body to increase joint laxity. Of course there is a very real need for this gradual loosening so that your pelvic joints are able to expand as the baby descends down the birth canal during labour. Stretching is a vital part of a balanced workout, and is often the 'treat' at the end of more arduous activity. Just be aware of your increased flexibility and make sure your stretching is gentle in nature. It is not a time to increase your flexibility, as this could set you up for permanent instability around the joints, pain or injury. A sensible approach is to stick to your normal range of movement when stretching and don't be tempted to push beyond that.

Whether pregnant or not, maintaining your flexibility will enhance your posture, reduce your chance of injury, reduce muscle soreness and tension, and maintain the range of motion of your joints. The muscle relaxation that follows stretching improves the circulation in your body. Stretching is a great rejuvenator and adds to an overall feeling of relaxation and wellbeing. All-over body stretching is recommended, but there are particular areas that you should stretch during the second trimester to lengthen potentially tight muscles due to your changing shape and posture: both lower and upper regions of your back, and your chest, shoulders and hip flexors.

The best time to slot in stretching is after warming up and after cooling down. If you are attending yoga, Pilates or specific stretching classes, tell the instructor that you are pregnant, and they should adapt the positions for you when required and give you safe stretching options.

Stretch technique

Check your form and alignment, then ease gently into the stretch position until you feel the muscle tighten with mild tension. Hold that position, breathe evenly. Maintain a static hold for 10–20 seconds, then ease off. Avoid bouncing while stretching, and avoid a style of stretching that involves contracting the muscle and then relaxing and pushing further into the stretch. This is referred to as 'proprioceptive neuromuscular facilitation' (PNF) and, while it is an effective way to increase your flexibility when you are not pregnant, it is potentially risky during pregnancy, as you could push beyond a safe range of movement and potentially injure yourself.

Stretches for the second trimester (Fig.6.17)

Using a Swiss ball provides a good tool for stretching against and alongside.

WITH BALL

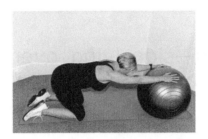

Double-arm pull-back off the ball.

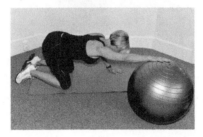

Chest and shoulder single-arm diagonals pull-back.

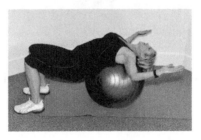

Chest opener—45° supine over ball.

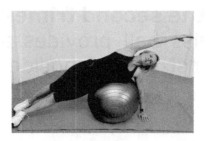

Side stretch—side lying over ball, full body extension, top arm over head.

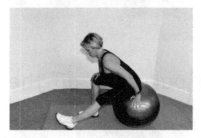

Hamstrings—sitting on ball, bending from hips, ankles flexed, one leg extended at a time.

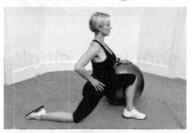

Hip flexor stretch—with one hand on ball.

WITH BALL

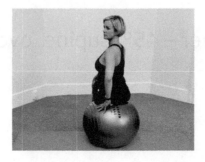

Sitting spine swivel—rotate upper body around and look behind.

STANDING

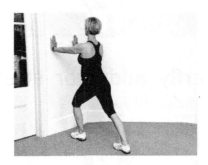

Calf stretch.

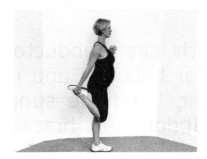

Standing quads stretch—one hand on wall.

FLOOR

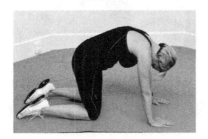

Cat stretch—on hands and knees, arching back up.

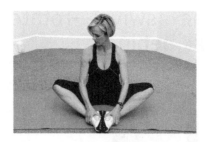

Sitting butterfly adductor stretch.

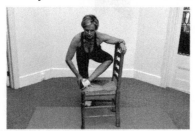

Standing with chair abductor stretch—hold onto the chair for balance, and lift one leg onto seat of the chair, bend the supporting leg and maintain an abdominal brace as you lean forward.

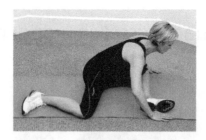

Option for hip area—sitting on the floor, knees bent at 90°, lean forward over front shin.

Pilates

This is an excellent choice as part of your exercise regime during this trimester, due to the focus on creating balance in the body, ideal posture and trunk stability. An added benefit for pregnant women is the Pilates emphasis on strengthening the pelvic floor and deep abdominals, and on an effective deep breathing technique, all of which are beneficial to you as your pregnancy progresses. You may wish to consider a prenatal Pilates class if you are a beginner, or, if you have been regularly participating during your first trimester, then ask the instructor what they recommend for this stage of pregnancy. It may be possible to continue on in your usual class (at least for the first half of this trimester), but with modifications to allow for your changing shape and body condition.

General modifications

⬤ Avoid lying on your tummy and, after 16 weeks, limit or avoid the time you spend lying on your back.

⬤ Limit abdominal movement to deep abdominal strengthening only, to avoid exacerbating any diastasis. (See Chapter 4 for more information on diastasis.)

⬤ Take care when moving on and off apparatus and when getting up and down from the floor.

⬤ Avoid wide leg positions to limit stress on your lower back and pelvis.

⬤ Limit the amount of time a position or contraction is held, and ensure you are not holding your breath. Modify the intensity of effort you put into stretching moves, making sure you only stretch within your normal range of flexibility and not beyond.

● Some moves may involve holding a position for a sustained amount of time; as your pregnancy progresses, limit the length of time you hold muscle contractions, and also consider gradually decreasing the number of repetitions.

Remember Pilates doesn't contribute to cardiovascular fitness, which is important to maintain, so make sure it is part of a balanced exercise programme. The skills you learn now in Pilates can help you minimise or avoid back pain for the remainder of your pregnancy, and will give you a head-start in easing your body back into shape after the birth.

Yoga

If morning sickness or other pregnancy complications have limited the type and amount of exercise you were able to do during the first trimester, then beginner or prenatal yoga is a good activity to either introduce or resume during the second trimester. Make sure you advise the instructor of your stage of pregnancy and if you have any back pain or joint issues they need to be aware of. Many women find this combination of both mind and body exercise, through a blend of flexibility, strength and relaxation practices, a balanced and rewarding experience during pregnancy. Yoga teaches you to tune in and listen to your body—this heightened sense of awareness has positive flow-on effects for you not only during pregnancy, but for your wellbeing in life in general. Learning to control the breath is an integral part of yoga, and many women find this skill useful during the early part of labour to help with relaxation and pain control.

If you are new to yoga and in your second trimester, then a mainstream class is likely to be too intense, so look for a specific prenatal yoga class. These classes are a great way of meeting other mums-to-be. For experienced yogis, it is a good idea to now switch to a prenatal class so that the poses and instruction are relevant to your changing and expanding body. Of course, classes are not the only way of doing yoga. Other ways of participating are through reading yoga books or following a yoga DVD, though it is preferable to have some experience already if you choose these options. For beginners, the best introduction is to practise under the watchful eye and guidance of an instructor.

For the best products, ask around and get recommendations from other mothers who have used them with success, or ask a qualified yoga instructor who may be able to advise you on what to buy.

General modifications

● The usual cautions for stretching while pregnant apply—only work within your usual range of movement, and do not be tempted or encouraged to push further or deeper into stretches—as due to your increased joint and ligament laxity (due to pregnancy hormones) you could injure yourself. Stretch and hold positions only to the point of mild tension, not pain, and as your pregnancy progresses decrease the length of time you hold a particular pose, around 10–20 seconds is adequate.

● Yoga positions have a definite focus on good posture, but in particular be aware of drawing in and bracing your abdominals, zipping up your pelvic floor muscles, and achieving alignment of neutral spine by tucking your tailbone under slightly to avoid over-arching your lower back.

● Avoid poses that require you to lie for an extended period on your back from approximately 16 weeks, due to the risk of supine hypotensive syndrome.

● Make space for your baby bump with any bending forwards or twisting moves. It is important not to compress the baby at all, so decrease the range of any twisting moves and try turning more from your shoulders rather than from your hips. Make space when bending forwards by taking a slightly wider stance. If you have hip, back or pubic symphysis problems, avoid taking your legs too far apart when either standing or sitting.

⬤ Many yoga poses require balance, which can be even more challenging during pregnancy due to your changing and altered centre of gravity. Use the wall or a chair to give you added support.

⬤ Avoid lying on your tummy, jumping into or out of poses, any rapid breathing or holding of the breath, and back bends. Either avoid or get instruction on how to modify inversions and abdominal work.

⬤ If in doubt, leave it out.

Dear Diary—Morning bunny

I've always been a bit of a morning bunny, but now with being pregnant the morning is definitely my glory time. I've noticed that by early evening I'm fading fast and I'm hitting the pillow by 9pm. Not exactly a bag of fun—but again I'm listening to my body. Oh, and my joints have started clicking, particularly my hips. After sitting for an hour or so I go to get up and there's often a loud click. It doesn't hurt, but it's a bit disconcerting. It's not just an age thing, although I definitely click more now that I'm in my forties! That clicking tells me my joints and ligaments are loosening up due to increased levels of the hormone relaxin (a name that really says what it does). I have also noticed from time to time a tooth will feel wobbly. It's weird to have spontaneous loosening of previously intact structures. I also had my big toe joint ache for two days for no good reason at all. I now know to act as a passive observer with these wobbles and niggles as they seem to spontaneously revert after just a few days. Crazy random pregnancy side-effects!

Two home workouts

Each is of approximately 40–50 minutes' duration. The first is a purely muscle-toning workout covering all the main muscle groups. The second is a cross-training workout, incorporating a combination of cardiovascular exercise with some strength training and stretching.

Remember that variety is the key, so intersperse these workouts at home with other activities that you enjoy. See the options mentioned earlier for other cardiovascular exercise or group fitness classes.

What you will need

Space

An area to work out in of about 2 metres square. If it's fine weather you might want to consider doing some of the exercises outside.

Equipment

A towel or a mat. If you haven't already bought one, then purchase a stretchy band or flex band/tube to provide some resistance for strength training. The bands are made of rubber, so keep them out of direct sunlight to preserve their integrity. They are not expensive and can be purchased at sporting goods stores or online. They come in different sizes and resistance levels; you may wish to purchase a couple to have both a light and a medium resistance. Some designs are tubing that has adjustable handles so you can alter length. This sort of equipment is a great tool for home workouts; they are easy to use and very portable. Other names that the bands are sold under include latex resistance, aerobic bands or resistance tubes.

Workout 1: Toning at home

With each exercise: remember to zip up your pelvic floor muscles and brace your abdominals to provide good lower back support and strong core stabilisation throughout.

Beginner level: 1 set of each exercise (after a few sessions you can increase to 2 sets).

Previously active and fit prior to pregnancy: 2–3 sets, completing each exercise in a slow and controlled manner so you feel the exertion but not exhaustion.

1 Pelvic tilts

Muscles used: abdominals and core stabilisers.

Key points: In standing, adopt a neutral spine position and tuck your tailbone under, curling your pubic bone towards your ribs. Deep abdominal brace as you tilt, then return to neutral. This is a great back pain reliever. If you have lower back ache, then a set of these pelvic tilts can really help alleviate the strain on your pelvis and lower back. You can also do some gentle pelvic tilts on the Swiss ball.

1 set: 15. Rhythm is 2 seconds tuck under, 2 seconds release back.

2 Smooth squats

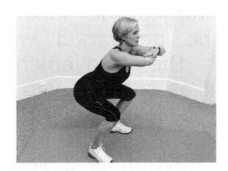

Fig.6.18

Muscles used: front and back of thigh, butt and back. An added bonus to this exercise is that it strengthens the muscles often used in labour. The squatting position opens up the pelvic area an extra 10%. It makes sense to strengthen the muscles that are required for squatting now, to possibly make your job a little easier later on! The squat must be performed with precision, and the slower the better. Consciously think of squeezing and tightening your buttocks when you stand up each time: imagine a $100 note between your butt cheeks that you don't want someone else to grab away!

Key points: Your feet are slightly wider than hip-distance apart. Bend at the knees and hips. Keep your back straight and tilt forward slightly at the hips, as if going to sit down on a chair. Squat until thighs are parallel to floor, then smoothly rise back up again. When down in the squat position, check the alignment of your

290

knees: they should point in line with the toes, but not extend beyond them. Turn your toes out more to target the inner thighs. This exercise can be performed with just body weight. Keep the movement slow and continuous, and as soon as you straighten the legs begin the next squat with no pause in between.

1 set: 20. Rhythm is 2 seconds down, 2 seconds up.

3 Standing one-leg knee-bends

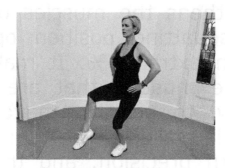

Fig.6.19

Muscles used: front and back of thigh, plus butt muscles with specific emphasis on lateral hip stability.

Key points: Get your balance standing on one leg and then lift your knee up to 90°. Make sure your knee is tracking directly forward over your toe as you bend and straighten, and not flaring in or out. Equally important is to not let the hip of your standing leg sway out to the side. Hitching up the bent-knee hip slightly can help with this.

1 set: 10 repetitions each leg. Rhythm is 2 seconds down, 2 seconds up.

4 Butt-lifts—bridging on ball

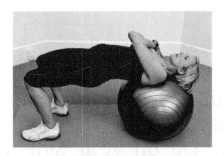

Fig.6.20

Muscles used: core, legs, gluteals.

Key points: Sit on top of the ball, and then let it roll up your back until your body weight is supported through your upper back (the ball will be between your shoulder blades). Your head and neck stays resting comfortably on the ball, your back is curved around the ball, and your hips are lowered. Your feet should be parallel, hip-distance apart, wider if you need more stability. Now squeeze your butt muscles and lift both hips evenly up towards horizontal, hold for 5 seconds, then lower down again.

1 set: 20. Rhythm is 2 seconds down, hold and squeeze 5 seconds, 2 seconds lower.

5 Side-lying leg-lifts

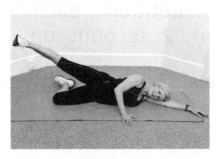

Fig.6.21

Muscles used: gluteals—specifically the gluteus medius.

Key points: Lie on your side with your hips stacked vertically. Bend the bottom knee for stability, then lift and lower the upper leg directly up and down.

1 set: 20 each side. Rhythm is 2 seconds up, 2 seconds down.

6 Press-ups

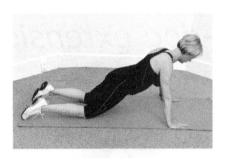

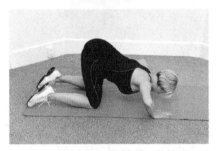

Fig.6.22

Muscles used: chest, tricep, abdominals, back.

Key points: from the second trimester, do half-press-ups or modified press-ups with the knees closer in towards your hands. Switch on your core muscles and brace your abdominals to maintain a straight back, and don't sag in the middle. Your hands are positioned slightly wider than your shoulders, knees about 20 centimetres apart. Lower your chest slowly to almost touch the floor, then press up to full elbow extension, but don't 'lock' the joint. To modify this half-press-up, bring your knees further in under your hips.

1 set: 15. Rhythm is 2 seconds down, 2 seconds up.

7 Hunting-dog extensions

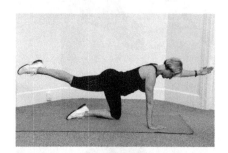

Fig.6.23

Muscles used: core stabilisers, back extensors, shoulder and butt.

Key points: Start on your hands and knees in the four-point position, spine neutral, abdominals braced, head and neck in line with the spine, and pelvic floor zipped up. Slide the opposite hand and leg out and extend them away from the body, lifting them up to almost horizontal, hold for 3–5 seconds, then slowly lower and return to the starting position. Keep your hips parallel to the floor and maintain a strong core region so you don't sag in the mid-region. Keep the movement slow and controlled.

1 set: Alternate 5 on each side

8 Triangle tricep extensions with flex band to provide resistance

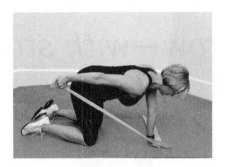

Fig.6.24

Muscles used: back of arm—triceps.

Key points: Get into the three-point kneeling position, with your left hand towards the middle so that your two knees and hand are the three points of a triangle. Distribute your body weight evenly between your three supporting limbs. Zip up your pelvic floor muscles, brace your deep abdominals, and keep your back flat. Secure the flex band or tube under your left hand (approximately half to a third of the way along its length) and take the shortest end in the right hand, lifting your upper arm level and parallel with your trunk. Lock it in there with elbow bent at 90°, now extend your hand up to horizontal as you stretch the band. At full extension, your thumb faces towards the floor and your little finger is facing towards the ceiling. Adjust the length of the band so that you can just reach horizontal. Make the up and down movement slow, controlled and continuous.

1 set: 12 on each side. Rhythm is 2 seconds down, 2 seconds up.

9 Seated row—with stretchy band/tube

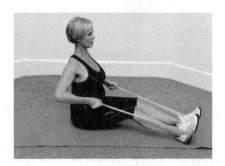

Fig.6.25

Muscles used: mid-back, biceps.

Key points: Sit with your legs extended (you can have a slight 10° bend in your knees if you find full leg extension difficult). Place the middle of the band around the arches of both feet, grip the band at about knee-level, then brace your abdominals, elevate the spine, keeping your back in neutral position, and pull both hands evenly towards your lower ribcage, squeezing your shoulder blades together. Don't raise your shoulders; keep them pressed down throughout.

1 set: 15. Rhythm is 2 seconds in, 2 seconds release.

10 Lateral raise—double-arm

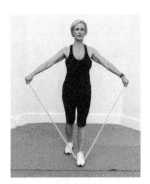

Fig.6.26

Muscles used: shoulder girdle.

Key points: Have the band running under your feet and up either side of your body, and stand with a wider-than-hip-distance-apart stance. Arms relaxed by your sides. Lift both arms out and up as far as you can towards horizontal, pause at the top, then slowly lower them down. Adjust your stance slightly wider or narrower to increase the resistance. The level you are able to lift up to the side may be determined by the length of your flex band. If the length is cutting your movement a bit short, try a split stance with one foot forward anchoring the band, as this should give you a bit more length of band to play with.

1 set: 12 repetitions. Rhythm is 2 seconds down, 2 seconds up.

11 Bicep curls—double-arm

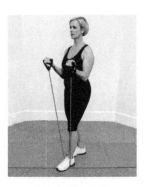

Fig.6.27

Muscles used: front of arm—biceps, forearm.

Key points: Secure the stretchy band under your feet, keeping your wrists locked in a neutral position, not flexed or extended. Curl both arms up to your shoulders and slowly lower them down to full extension, keeping the movement continuous. The down movement is just as important as the up movement for the strength of the muscle, so don't just let go at the top and rush the downwards phase of the movement—take your time and use all the counts. Keep your shoulders down and maintain a good upright posture throughout.

1 set: 12 repetitions. Rhythm is 2 seconds down, 2 seconds up.

12 Abdominals

A Abdominal lifts—in four-point kneeling

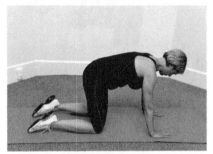

Fig.6.28

Starting position: On all fours with your hands under your shoulders and knees under your hips. Keep your elbows soft and back in a neutral position, and your head in line with your spine.

Action: Tilt your pelvis to neutral by contracting the deep abdominals, and on an exhale pull your belly button up towards your spine and hold the contraction for 5–10 seconds, breathing evenly. Note is it *not* a back arch. When performed correctly, your back should stay relatively flat. At the end of the contraction, relax your abdominals but don't push down or arch your back.

1 set: 10–15 repetitions.

B Core—four-point hover

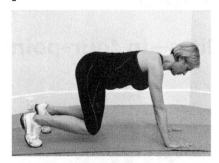

Fig.6.29

Starting position: Position yourself on your hands and knees. Keep your head in line with your spine, and look down at the floor. Maintain a neutral spine

Action: Draw in the abdominals and brace. Holding this position, on an exhale gently raise your knees just 5 centimetres off the floor, hold and hover there for 5–10 seconds, and then lower both knees to the floor. Avoid lifting too high or the exercise will become too easy. Don't hold your breath.

1 set: 10–15 repetitions.

C Core—side-lying half-plank

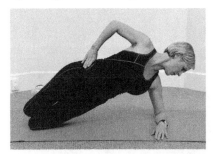

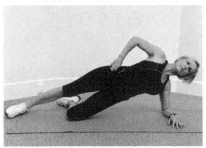

Fig.6.30

Starting position: Lie on your side, legs bent behind your body, your thighs and torso in line.

Action: Press down through your grounded elbow and forearm, and lift your hips up off the floor so that you have a straight body-line from your upper shoulder to your knees. Hold for 5–10 seconds, then lower. Do a set of 10, then roll over and do the same on the other side. If you wish to advance this exercise, extend the legs fully and hold your body straight from your feet to your bent elbow.

D Side crunches

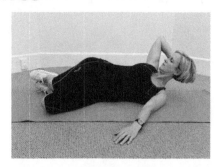

Fig.6.31

Starting position: Lie on your side, keeping your lower leg bent and extending your lower arm slightly in front of your body for stability. Put your other hand behind your head, supporting but not pulling up.

Action: Exhale as you lift the ribcage toward the hip bone, squeezing in the waistline, inhale and lower down.

1 set: 10–15 repetitions, roll over and complete a matching set on the other side.

13 Stretch

Complete a set of the stretches as illustrated under section entitled "Stretch technique". Congratulations, you're done! Drink a big glass of water.

Workout 2: Cross-training at home

* 30 minutes of cardiovascular training
* 30 minutes of strength training interspersed with stretching

Part 1

If you have been jogging throughout the first trimester, now is the time to ease off the intensity. A fast walk is preferable for the second trimester, and if your route entails hills then take your time walking up them. When you walk uphill you will naturally lean forward slightly, which can place extra stress on your lower back, so protect it by keeping your deep abdominals pulled in. Aim to have your RPE between 5 and 6 ('somewhat hard'). Walk easily for the first 5 minutes as a warm-up, then pick up the pace, swinging your arms. You should feel as if your heart rate and breathing rate have increased for the duration of 30 minutes, but you should not be puffing or out of breath. If you have home cardiovascular exercise equipment (such as a bike, treadmill, etc.), you could also choose to do a 30-minute session indoors.

Stretch

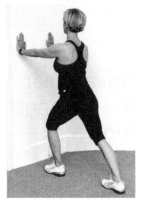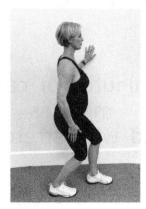

Fig.6.32

Complete Part 1 by doing both straight-knee and bent-knee calf stretches.

Part 2

You will already be warmed up from doing the cardiovascular component first, so now you can launch straight into the toning exercises. The programme is set out in superset style, which means you partner exercises together, alternating a set of each exercise. This will give you a time-efficient workout. For detailed descriptions of each of the muscles targeted and the action for each exercise, see the muscle-toning workout, above.

With each exercise: Remember to zip up your pelvic floor muscles and brace your abdominals to provide good lower back support and strong core stabilisation throughout.

1 Smooth squats and bridged butt-lifts and side-lying leg-lifts superset (legs and butt) with ball

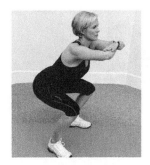

Fig.6.33

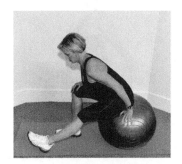

Fig.6.34

1x20 squats, 1x20 butt-lifts,
1x20 side leg-lifts each side—repeat. 1x20 squats, 1x20 butt-lifts,
1x20 side leg lifts each side.

Stretches x 2, alternate legs, hold for 10 seconds.

2 Half-press-ups and hunting-dog extensions superset (chest and back)

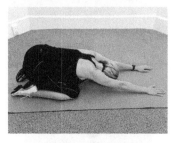

Fig.6.35

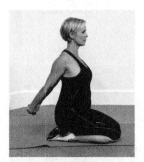

Fig.6.36

15 x press-ups, 3 x R then L arm plus leg extensions with 5-second hold,
15 x press-ups, 3 x R then L arm plus leg extensions with 5-second hold.

Stretches x 2, hold for 10 seconds.

3 Seated row/triangle tricep extensions, lateral raise (mid-back and arms) with flex band

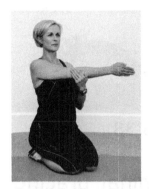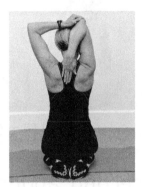

Fig.6.37

15 x seated rows, turnover into kneeling, 15 x tricep extensions on one side, 15 x seated rows, 15 x tricep extensions on other side.

Then 2 sets of 15 x lateral raises with 30-second rest in between sets.

Stretches x 2, hold for 10 seconds.

4 Abdominals (targeting deep abdominals and core)

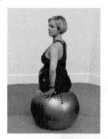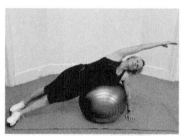

Fig.6.38

15x5-second abdominal bracing in four-point kneeling, 5 x four-point core hovers, 5–10 seconds each.

Then side half-plank holds, one on each side, hold for 20–30 seconds each, with good form and even breathing throughout.

Stretches x 2, hold for 10 seconds.

Congratulations, you're done!
Now have a big drink of water.

Key considerations for the second trimester

This stage of pregnancy is considered the most stable and is typically the most enjoyable. Early pregnancy discomforts of nausea, tiredness and breast tenderness have generally disappeared. It is also the time when real body expansion begins, but you are not yet so big that you feel cumbersome when moving around, so relax and relish this time. From the beginning of the second trimester, the baby has all its organs and systems in place and is now focused on growing. It is a great time to exercise, to maintain or gain some cardiovascular fitness that will stand you in good stead for the remainder of your pregnancy and beyond, to tone and strengthen those muscles that support good posture and provide relief from back and pelvic aches and pain. The work you put in now will also contribute to how quickly you recover after giving birth. A fit, healthy mum is certainly giving her baby a great head start.

Speaking from personal experience as a new mum in my forties, having some fitness resilience didn't eliminate the inevitable tiredness but it definitely made my post-birth recovery smoother and helped restore my energy levels more quickly.

Dear Diary—Breathless at 20 steps

Stairs are quite a challenge at present. It doesn't seem right that this extra basketball out front should result in me having to pause and catch my breath after one measly set of stairs, but that is exactly what happens. I can't stand any clothing that's vaguely snug-fitting around my bump. Pants have become a thing of the past unless they are super-stretchy tights or preggy-pants which finish below the bump and have a massive wide waistband of elastic. I did spend an extraordinary amount of time online looking for belt-extender gadgets. Only to bid and buy one online for about $10 and then find it was a pick-up in a far-off rural location that cost at least $10 petrol to retrieve. It's funny, I don't know if it's just me but I find I do get quite fixated on things at present; whether it's finishing off a task or getting my point across. I think as my tummy has expanded my tolerance has shrunk. I think I remember this happening last time. The good thing is most people afford pregnant women a little more latitude—just as well!

What's the ideal exercise regime?

If you are feeling great and your pregnancy is progressing normally, then include a mixed programme of cardiovascular exercise, strength training and stretching.

✳ **Beginners**—three times a week of 30 minutes of moderate exercise.

✳ **Experienced exercisers**—40–60 minutes a day most days of the week, at moderate intensity.

Here is a sample programme of what you could do over a period of seven days to ensure that your programme of regular, moderate exercise on most days of the week has balance and variety. It is intended as a guide only, as you need to figure out how to best incorporate regular exercise into your individual lifestyle so that it becomes an enhancement and not a stressor. Take the principles of balance, variety and moderation, and plan out a weekly regime that is both achievable and enjoyable for YOU. If you need help designing a programme, then talk to a qualified gym instructor who should be able to give you some ideas of how to structure your workouts to achieve your goals.

Suggested Weekly Plan

Monday *Cardio focus.* Walk, jog, or gym class that increases your heart rate, 30–60 minutes' duration, RPE 5–6.

Tuesday *Strength focus.* Modified strength training at the gym or using home toning workout, 45–60 minutes.

Wednesday *Core and stretch focus.* Pilates or yoga or Bare Essentials routine at home, including pelvic floor exercises, 30 minutes.

Thursday Day off.

Friday *Cardio focus.* Gym class or walking that increases your heart rate, 30–60 minutes' duration, RPE 5–6.

Saturday *Low-impact day.* Swimming or core exercises or Pilates or yoga, body balance class, 30–45 minutes.

Sunday *Strength focus day* or *optional day off* or *Bare Essentials routine.*

Key points

○ Keep communicating with your LMC about your exercise regime.

○ Stick to regular, moderate exercise with a modified intensity of about 5–6 RPE. Keep your heart rate no higher than approximately 140–160bpm.

○ In general, you should have decreased your exercise exertion by about 5–10% and modified the exercises you were doing during the first trimester.

○ As your body shape changes, pay extra care to good posture in sitting and standing, and increase your focus on strengthening those deep abdominals to provide support to your growing baby bump and lower back.

○ Prevent back pain and maintain pelvic stability by including regular hip-muscle exercises, such as side leg-lifts and standing single-leg balance exercises.

○ Listen to your body and reduce the exertion if you feel extra tired. It is important to stay fit during pregnancy, but not to the detriment of your overall wellbeing.

○ If you were planning to travel, this is a good time to do so, as your hormones have stabilised and you are 'showing' but are not restricted in movement.

○ Enjoy this 'blooming lovely' time!

√ Make your water-bottle your best friend, and increase your fluid intake for adequate hydration.

√ Avoid overheating, and modify your exercise in hot and humid environments.

√ Warm up and cool down slowly.

√ Do pelvic tilts regularly to relieve lower back strain.

√ Modify your abdominal exercises to account for a diastasis: no sit-ups, but yes to deep abdominals.

√ Don't overstretch, and make sure you promote pelvic stability with strengthening and standing balance exercises.

√ Eat either side of your workout, keeping healthy snacks in your handbag.

√ Get a good balance between rest and activity—ensure adequate time for both.

Chapter 7

The Third Trimester (28–40+ weeks)

The end is in sight

In just three months, give or take a few days, there will be a beautiful outcome to your pregnancy journey. They say there is nothing *certain* in life apart from death and taxes, but at 28 weeks pregnant there is certain inevitability to the impending arrival of 'a new son or daughter'. Preparing for the birth and preparing to bring your new baby home are naturally where your focus will be over these next few months, so how does exercise fit in?

During the third trimester, regular, moderate exercise still plays an important part in an uncomplicated pregnancy. A fit, healthy woman is more likely to take on the rigours of labour with a positive mental attitude, good body awareness and improved resilience. Exercise can also help alleviate the sort of pregnancy symptoms typical of this stage, like insomnia, swollen ankles and back ache. That said, it is also particularly important over these next 12 weeks to listen to your body and balance exercise with sufficient rest. Slowing down is normal. Increasing dramatically in size is normal, too. The baby will be packing on around 28 grams a day, and you can expect to see your weight increase by an average of 5 kilograms. Where you carry your weight shifts, too, with the baby riding lower down in the pelvis. You will be seeing your LMC frequently during this time, initially with fortnightly appointments, then closer to your due date it will be weekly, so make sure to communicate with them the sort of exercise you are undertaking.

Dear Diary—Up at night

Yay, I'm 28 weeks! But I still have a 30-week milestone in my head to reach, as that's when I reckon I'm in more of a 'safe zone' in case I have a very early delivery. Now baby just has to grow in size, and that's going to be interesting as my front bump already feels stretched tight and at maximum capacity. Peanut is measuring 30 weeks already, but evidently the scans are only a rough guide. I'm writing this in the early hours of the morning: it is 3am, the house is quiet. I hear a random tweet from a bird outside, it's obviously testing to see if dawn is anywhere near. It's not – I'm sure of that! The reason I'm up again in the wee small hours is indigestion which still wakes me up. I'm getting lots of wind and discomfort. The obstetrician says that the internal gut sphincters that normally keep everything down soften during pregnancy and therefore aren't as tightly shut, so that's why you get reflux, or 'back draft' as I prefer to call it. Hubby is upstairs in the spare room, a self-imposed exile to the spare bed thanks to my ongoing snoring issues. Okay, I'd better try to get back to sleep now, it's only been a one-hour interlude. I guess it's a taste of being up in the middle of the night once Peanut arrives.

Changes continue

Changes to baby

From 28 weeks the baby's systems are all functioning and the focus is predominantly on baby building body size by laying down fat stores. So make sure you are eating a good balanced diet with plenty of protein. The baby's kidneys are working, so they pass urine which is removed via the placenta. The baby's hearing is now well developed, with some women finding that loud or rhythmic music evokes a response with increased activity in the womb. The baby now has active and restful periods, which often occurring at similar times each day. This sort of activity patterning can even continue after birth. If your baby was a real 'kicker' in the mornings in the womb, then you could be in for a very alert 'morning baby'.

Changes to mother

During the first two trimesters your circulating blood volume has been gradually increasing to what now amounts to almost double. Your heart rate must therefore correspondingly increase to pump this extra fluid around your body and to your baby. This increased blood flow can give a healthy glow to your appearance, but can also add to the pregnancy side-effects of swollen lower limbs and ankles. Some women will also be genetically predisposed to varicose veins. This is where the superficial leg veins become swollen and painful due to pregnancy hormones acting on walls of the veins, making them less effective at pumping blood back to the heart. Regular exercise and maintaining muscle tone can help increase circulation which can lessen some of this blood pooling. Other tips are to avoid standing still or sitting for long periods, and avoid crossing your legs. You may wish to use support tights, as the pressure can provide some relief; just make sure you remove them before exercising.

Increased circulation can also cause nasal congestion: that feeling of a stuffy blocked nose. You may even think you are getting a cold. Talk to your doctor about suitable ways to get some relief (inhalations, etc.), but rest assured it does disappear after birth. You may also get bouts of feeling hot and flushed as your body temperature increases slightly. Your baby is doing a great job as an internal hot-water bottle!

Remember back to the first trimester when you probably felt like your bladder was the size of a thimble and you were endlessly going to the toilet? Well that familiarity with the little room is about to return, but this time the trigger is the weight of your growing baby pushing down on your bladder. Do not decrease your fluid intake—it is important that you are adequately hydrated for your baby's sake. Just add your frequent bathroom visits to the 'oh well' list of pregnancy idiosyncrasies.

Dear Diary—Extra bits

I have noticed in the past week a handful of skin tags appearing, on my upper chest area and breasts. At first I did a minor freak-out, thinking they were some form of skin cancer, but no they're purely freckle-sized little skin blobs. Actually the pregnancy websites describe them as 'small, soft, flesh coloured hanging growths'—fabulous! Evidently they are quite common in pregnancy, and come about probably because of hyperactive growth of a superficial layer of skin caused by hormonal changes. They're not painful and are completely benign. If they hang around after birth I think I'll get them removed by a professional, either with liquid nitrogen freezing or cauterising, as that seems to be the normal way of dealing with these visitors. Yet another minor weirdness due to pregnancy that you can't do anything about.

Exercise and side-effects

General fatigue levels do naturally increase during this time. You are heavier, larger and carrying around more weight than you have before, so you are getting a workout just participating in your normal life. Exercise intensity and the duration of your workouts will need to be adjusted. If you are sleeping relatively well and feeling fine, then try to keep to 30–60 minutes most days of the week. But always remember, a day or two off to revitalise your energy levels is absolutely fine. A good balance of rest and exercise is important. Some days you might just run through a series of stretches or do a gentle walk and that will feel enough. Other days you may feel up to doing your usual exercising routine. While there is no hard-and-fast rule, a good rule of thumb is for every hour you spend exercising you should spend at least half that time resting, preferably with your feet up.

What the research says

• Continuing or starting a regular exercise programme does not increase a woman's chances of either rupturing her membranes or going in to labour early.

• Lots of weight-bearing exercise right until term (38–40 weeks) does increase a woman's chances of delivering shortly before her due date by about 50%.

• Non-weight-bearing exercise does not alter the timing of labour, and the same is true for women who either continue weight-bearing exercise at a substantially reduced level or cease exercising completely.

Source: James F Clapp III MD, *Exercising Through Your Pregnancy.*

Keeping it all in perspective

Some women breeze through their third trimester trouble-free, others will be very aware of getting heavier and larger and find their movements restricted, while some may struggle with one or more pregnancy symptom. Each woman's journey is unique. The considerations listed below are not an exhaustive or prescriptive list. Please don't assume that you will necessarily get all or any of these third trimester ailments. However, if you do feel the effects of some of these potential barriers to fitness, then hopefully the tips to follow will equip you to better cope, allowing you to modify your exercise regime to maintain a suitable level of activity.

Nausea, heartburn and indigestion

Just when the memory of first trimester morning sickness was fading, you could find it returns as you enter these final few months. Some women unfortunately may experience nausea and even vomiting again during this stage. It can be partly due to hormones again, but also playing a part is the baby itself, with its sheer size putting pressure on your internal organs which can upset the stomach. Heartburn (or acid reflux) can also occur because of the combination of hormones relaxing the valve between the stomach and oesophagus, and baby size impinging on your stomach. A small amount of stomach acid can seep upwards into your oesophagus, giving a burning sensation behind the breastbone. Indigestion is also common during the second and third trimesters. Again, pregnancy hormones act to slow down the muscle action that takes place in digestion, slowing the whole process and leaving you feeling very full, bloated or gassy.

Tips to help with nausea, heartburn and indigestion

* Eat smaller meals but more frequently throughout the day, and don't bolt your food. Consider having five or six smaller meals rather than three larger meals.

* Stay sitting upright for at least an hour after you eat.

* Avoid greasy, fatty or spicy foods. Other foods that can be problematic include onions, garlic, chocolate, and coffee or caffeine-containing drinks, as well as certain medications.

* Avoid drinking large amounts of fluid with your meal, but instead drink in between meals whenever possible.

* Talk to your LMC or pharmacist about suitable antacid formulations that are suitable to take during pregnancy.

Insomnia

This is very common during this late phase of pregnancy. Maybe its Mother Nature's way of getting you familiar with less sleep or broken sleep to ease you into the newborn baby routine. Well, that's what I kept telling myself as I stared endlessly at the bedroom ceiling. It is particularly frustrating, as during the very stage when you feel you need good-quality sleep, you are ending up short-changed.

What to do

Moderate exercise can help with sleeplessness, provided it is not in the evening before you are about to go to bed. Allow sufficient time to wind down after exercising before you lie down. If you think you are staying awake because your mind is buzzing with ideas or worries (or in my case 'to do lists'), then have a piece of paper and a pen by your bedside and write your thoughts down so you can mentally let go. If you have practised any relaxation techniques in yoga, Pilates or perhaps at antenatal classes, this is a good time to put them to use. Just concentrating on deep breathing, systematically contracting and relaxing the large muscle groups, or persuading your partner to give you a massage might do the trick. Also 'set the scene'. Begin your wind-down routine several hours prior to bed. Try any or all of these suggestions: have a warm bath, lower your stimulation levels, read a book, or have a warm milk drink.

Braxton Hicks contractions

These are preparation for labour contractions that occur with a tightening of the muscles of the uterus, possibly accompanied by mild period-type pains. They are increasingly common in the third trimester, but can occur even a few months into the first trimester. Many women experience these Braxton Hicks contractions (named after the scientist who discovered them in 1872), and you'll be pleased to know they do have a purpose. Like a mini dress-rehearsal, they actually help your body prepare for labour. The uterus contracts as it will do in labour, but to a much lesser extent. They generally last between one and two minutes, and should be uncomfortable rather than painful. They can occur quite randomly, but certain activities commonly trigger them, including: the baby moving around; heavy exercise or lifting; touching your abdomen; sexual intercourse; and dehydration.

Even though they are called 'practice contractions', they can easily be distinguished from proper labour contractions which show a pattern of increasing in intensity, increasing in frequency and being clearly painful. Experiencing Braxton Hicks contractions is not a reason to stop exercising; they are more just a nuisance. They are not an indicator of when you will begin real labour, so if possible just take a pause until they subside and then go about your regular routine.

What to do

Most women will just take a pause when they occur and rest for a short time until they pass, but sometimes a change of movement can also help alleviate discomfort. Make sure you stay hydrated. Lying down on your left side may ease them. Try emptying your bladder. If they are getting more intense towards the end of your third trimester, try a few slow, deep breaths to relax your body.

Carpal tunnel syndrome

The increase in total blood volume that builds during pregnancy of approximately 40%, combined with the effect of pregnancy hormones, mean some women are prone to excess fluid retention. The wrist has a relatively narrow passage (the carpal tunnel) for the main nerve to pass through that supplies the thumb and index finger with sensation. If there is extra fluid build-up in this area the nerve can become squashed, which causes tingling, numbness and pain or stiffness in the wrist and hand. It can occur on one side or both, prenatally and postnatally. The typical time for symptoms to occur is around 24 weeks when fluid retention is particularly common. Interestingly, research shows that women between the ages of 30 and 60 have the highest incidence of carpal tunnel syndrome, and pregnant women in the 30- to 40-year-old age group have a higher risk of potentially developing the condition.

What to do

If you experience carpal tunnel syndrome, then avoid exercising positions where your weight is taken through a flexed wrist position. Gripping may also cause discomfort. Keep your wrists in a neutral position (not bent or flexed) when lifting weights or doing resistance work. You may have to modify your exercise choice to things where your wrists won't be placed under strain, like swimming or walking. If using a computer keyboard is uncomfortable, try using a wrist pad to give extra support, and check your sitting position to ensure you have good ergonomics. Wrist splints (although uncomfortable to wear) may also provide some relief at night. Discuss this with your LMC and seek their advice on appropriate treatment.

Lower back pain, sacroiliac pain and symphysis pubis dysfunction

During the third trimester the strain on your pelvis and lower back is further increased due to the rapid gain of weight and size by both baby and mother. You may also notice your baby bump is descending compared with the second trimester when it sat higher up. This is completely normal, but the physical effect on the body is that your centre of gravity moves forward, bringing a tendency to over-arch the lower back. Increased weight and altered posture, combined with softening of ligaments due to the action of the pregnancy hormone relaxin, means you are at increased risk of pelvic instability. The usually firm non-moveable fibrous joints at the rear between your sacrum and pelvis, and at the front of the pelvic ring (pubic symphysis), become slightly mobile, and this can cause considerable pain and discomfort. Scans have revealed some women have gaps at their pubic symphysis joint of around 4 millimetres with some even extending to 9 millimetres. The pain tends to be made worse by walking and by uneven weight distribution; for example, if you stand on one leg. Any strain or jerk may also stress the weakened joints. Getting out of the bath becomes difficult or impossible without help, and getting in and out of cars or seats can be problematic.

What to do

If you are suffering from this sort of pain, then weight-bearing exercise should cease. However, water-based exercise may be achievable. Minimise walking up or down stairs, and reduce lifting and carrying whenever possible. Avoid movements where you are separating your legs, like getting in and out of the car, climbing over gates, or stretching positions with your legs apart. Rest is important, but so too is gentle exercise, so try water-buoyancy-assisted activities like aqua jogging or swimming (but specifically not breaststroke). Exercises that strengthen and maintain core and hip stability are worth doing to provide as much pelvic support as possible—focus on the deep abdominals, back and buttock muscles. You may find wearing a rigid or non-rigid pelvic support belt provides some relief as well.

Many women who are pain-free before labour find the actual birth process ends up straining their pubic symphysis joint and they experience these symptoms postnatally. For most women, once the pregnancy hormones diminish after birth, the ligaments tighten up and the pain usually subsides. However, patience is necessary as it could take days or weeks. If you are experiencing this sort of pain and discomfort during or after pregnancy, discuss this condition with your LMC or doctor, who may refer you to a physiotherapist specialising in women's health for further advice and treatment.

High blood pressure

Your blood pressure will be regularly monitored by your LMC during your increasingly regular visits during this trimester. Typically it drops during the second trimester and returns to normal during the third trimester. A normal reading is less than 140/90 (140mmHg systolic over 90mmHg diastolic). A high reading is 140/90 or greater.

If your LMC notices that your blood pressure is abnormally high, they may suggest you modify or rest from exercise for a few days to let it settle down. A retest will determine whether further intervention is needed. High blood pressure can be a serious problem, as it reduces blood flow to the baby, restricting growth. Don't hesitate to contact your LMC if you think you have high blood pressure that hasn't yet been detected.

Pre-eclampsia

This is one of the reasons why your blood pressure is carefully monitored throughout pregnancy. Pre-eclampsia is a high blood pressure disorder that occurs in 5–10% of pregnant women, and is also revealed by protein in the urine and abnormal swelling of hands, face or legs. It is more common in pregnant women over the age of 35 and typically occurs after the twentieth week. Pre-eclampsia is potentially dangerous to both mother and baby. While exercising can reduce your risk of *getting* pre-eclampsia, once you have it then it is likely your LMC will recommend rest.

Stress incontinence

Even with fastidious attention to exercising your pelvic floor muscles, the sheer weight of the baby pushing down on your bladder during the final few weeks of pregnancy can cause mild stress incontinence, with just a small amount of leakage when you cough, laugh or strain. Remind yourself to be even more vigilant with pelvic floor exercises, and make sure you get on to exercising them (even if it is only a barely perceptible flicker) the very next day after delivering.

Shortness of breath

Even if you are fit and active, by the third trimester you are carrying a heavy and awkward load, and the pressure of the expanding uterus on your respiratory system can cause shortness of breath even with mild exertion. Always exercise moderately, and if you find yourself puffing and panting, slow down, pause, or stop and rest.

Leg cramps

Cramps typically occur in the calf muscles and often in the middle of the night. Moderate weight-bearing exercise can help reduce the incidence of cramp by improving circulation through the lower limbs.

What to do

No one knows why leg cramps occur more frequently during the second and third trimesters, but if you do suffer from them then try these cramp preventers and relievers:

✓ Stretch your calf muscles following exercising and before you go to bed.

✓ Avoid standing or sitting with your legs crossed for long periods of time.

✓ Improve leg circulation by rotating your ankles and wiggling your toes frequently.

✓ Try a warm bath and massage your calves before bedtime.

✓ Ensure you are adequately hydrated.

✓ For immediate relief when you have a cramp, stretch your calf muscle by straightening your leg and flexing your ankle, toes up towards your knee. It may be uncomfortable at first, but it should ease the cramping sensation. Take a walk around and massage or rub the muscle.

✓ Take calcium and magnesium supplements, but always discuss supplements with your LMC first.

Stitch

It is quite common during pregnancy to get the stitch when exercising—an ache or sharp pain felt close to the ribs and usually on one side. There are several reasons that it could occur during this stage of pregnancy: the weight of the baby pulling down internal organs, abdominal stretching, or the baby may be pushing up into the ribs.

What to do

Try side stretching, taking your arm up and over your head and gently bend to the side, so you increase the gap between your hip and ribs on the painful side. A maternity support belt may also provide some support and ease symptoms. Buoyancy-assisted exercising in the pool rather than weight-bearing activities may also prevent the onset of stitch.

Good breast and pelvis support

Comfort when exercising during this stage of pregnancy makes all the difference. Your breasts will be noticeably larger, and the milk-producing areas (alveoli) are now becoming full developed as they prepare for breastfeeding. Towards the end of the third trimester you may even notice small amounts of milk (colostrum) being produced, so you may decide to wear breast pads, particularly when exercising. The key with support of the breasts at this stage is to secure them firmly against your chest, and the best way to do that is by wearing two firm sports bras, one on top of the other.

To support the pelvis the key is upward lift to minimise the downward pressure of gravity. A range of pelvic support belts are available under various names—prenatal cradle, maternity belt, etc. Some are made from rigid material, some are flexible. You should be able to buy one from a retail store or online. They are usually wide elasticised material with velcro at either end, and they circle snugly around the lower back and pelvis, providing mild compression and support to the pelvic bones, helping with stability. This sort of belt should not replace good core abdominal strengthening exercises, as you can't always wear the belt. But if you find during the latter stages of pregnancy, while exercising or in general, that you are feeling aches and strain in your lower back and pelvic region, then you may find a support belt provides some relief.

Dear Diary—A moan and a craving

This sounds terribly ungrateful, especially after all the trials and tribulations we've been through to even get pregnant, but by this stage of pregnancy I'm finding there are symptoms that are just truly tiresome. Rolling over to get out of bed and getting out of a chair or off the couch are now all manoeuvred in a different way. Not to mention the hassle of getting up in the early hours of the morning to go to the loo. Okay, that's the moan over. It's just good to get it off my chest, now I can go back to being thankful with every cell in my body that we are where we are. Oh, I have discovered a craving—chocolate Paddle Pop ice-blocks. I had to go and buy an extra box at the supermarket last night to make sure we didn't run out. I like to have at least one, sometimes two, at night. A little ice-cold treat—which suits two purposes: it's humid and hot this month, and I'm meant to be consuming more calcium at present to support baby's growth. I know a Paddle Pop is a very long stretch when it comes to containing a decent calcium-containing product, but it reminds me to have yogurt and milk, too. Fresh fruit and low-fat but high-calcium milk smoothies are another favourite of mine at the moment.

Care and posture

Now is the time when you should really be aware and mindful of your posture. Remember, maintaining good posture in standing and sitting will benefit you in many ways, including: less back ache, less pelvic pain, better breathing capacity, and a feeling of overall wellbeing. So here is a timely reminder from the posture advice given in Chapter 4. As your pregnancy progresses, what was a small lower back curve becomes increasingly exaggerated, with your tummy extending forwards and increasing in weight. This can put extra strain on your already stretched abdominals and more stress on your spine. Heavier, fuller breasts can cause you to round your shoulders and slump forwards, which in turn forces your chin to jut forward, placing extra stress down the back of your neck (cervical spine). Due to your increasing weight you will probably stand with your feet wider apart for balance, and that in itself can apply different stresses to the hips and lower back. Avoid standing still for long periods, as the longer you are in the upright position the more likely you are to sag into bad posture and in essence 'hang on your ligaments'. Whenever possible take the weight off your feet and sit in a chair with good back support. Standing still for extended periods also causes sluggish circulation and the potential pooling of fluids in your lower limbs and feet. If you *have* to stand still, then rise up and down occasionally on your toes; this pumps your calf muscles and assists with circulation. Avoid or minimise lifting whenever possible. If you do need to lift, make sure your deep abdominals are drawn in and braced, keep the load close to you, and let your legs take the strain rather than your back. Walk your feet around rather than lifting and twisting.

Standing smart when pregnant

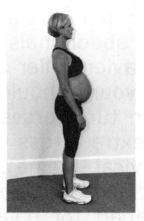

Fig.7.1

Working down the body from your head to your feet, let's run through the postural alignment for good standing posture. Chin tucked so that your eyes are looking forward, slide your chin back towards your spine (retraction), shoulders down and back. Tuck your tailbone slightly under, with your feet hip-distance apart, and your knees soft and not locked into extension. Finally, lengthen through your mid-section by extending the gap between your ribs and hips. Try imagining a plumb-line attached to the very apex of your skull which is gently pulling you up a few centimetres.

Sitting smart when pregnant

Beware of sitting evenly on your sit bones. The process of elongating and stacking your spine correctly starts right from the sit bones and continues all the way up to the top of your neck. Be aware of maintaining the small natural curve in your lower back. You can try using a small pillow, lumbar roll or rolled-up towel to help you maintain that natural lower back curve, and make sure you shuffle your buttocks to the back of the seat when sitting. Then 'sit tall' by lifting your ribcage away from your pelvis, creating a sense of elongation in your mid-region. Finally, roll your shoulders back and down.

Research on exercising during the third trimester

Some mothers choose to decrease or stop exercising in the third trimester, perhaps due to their increasing size, just being plain tired, or thinking that it will be too stressful on the baby. The research suggests that continuing is beneficial, if you are able to without complications. Studies have shown that stopping exercise late in pregnancy results in a larger baby with more body fat, whereas continuing exercise right up until term resulted in babies with normal birth weights but with less body fat.

In particular, continuing with weight-bearing exercising, like power-walking or low-impact aerobics, right up until full term does increase the chance of delivering a few days or possibly even as much as a week before your due date. For most pregnant women, who by 37 or 38 weeks are heartily sick of being the size of a whale, this is not necessarily a bad thing. Conversely, non-impact forms of exercise, like swimming, or reducing the amount of exercise overall in the third trimester does not seem to affect or bring forward the timing of delivery.

Source: James F Clapp III MD, *Exercising Through Your Pregnancy.*

Dear Diary—Confession of a muffin stuff-up

You know how pregnant women are routinely checked at approx 28 weeks for gestational diabetes? Well I did a dumb thing. I booked in for my blood test at 4pm (at the end of the working day) and then proceeded to have lunch at about 1pm (a sandwich) and then a muffin snack at about 2pm. As I now know, it's not the best lead-up to having your blood sugar checked and measured, because you are pre-loaded with sugar thanks to the sticky muffin.

They test you over the period of an hour, giving you a very sweet drink to consume in the first 10 minutes, then they compare baseline blood sugars with how your body has processed the sugary drink. With added sugar in my system already, I rated very high. High enough that my obstetrician said I needed to do a phase two test. This time it involved fasting beforehand, another blood test and then a further wait and repeat blood test. It came out normal.

Tip for newbie mums-to-be: do the first blood test first thing in the morning, not once you have nibbled and snacked your way through the day like I did. Duh! I could have done without being stuck with needles a second time. You live and learn.

Cardiovascular exercise

Having established that continued exercise is good for you, remember that if you experience any of the following symptoms during exercise, simply stop the activity and discuss the situation with your LMC:

* excessive shortness of breath
* headache or dizziness
* pain—in particular chest or abdomen pain
* nausea or vomiting
* vaginal bleeding
* contractions
* deep back or pubic pain
* cramping in the lower abdomen
* sudden swelling of the hands, face and ankles
* unusual change in the baby's movements—usually a marked decrease
* amniotic fluid leakage.

Suitable third-trimester cardiovascular exercise

General exercise tips

Any activity should be limited to your level of comfort. Walking and swimming are both excellent exercise choices that can be done every day. Ensure you do a gentle warm-up of at least 5–10 minutes and spend a similar time cooling down at the conclusion of your workout. Keep your exercise intensity now to around 4-5 RPE (rate of perceived exertion—see Chapter 1), which can be described as 'fairly light' to 'somewhat hard'. Dress in layers to avoid overheating, and ensure adequate hydration by frequently sipping water. You may find having a small snack prior to or after exercising helps maintain a good level of blood sugar and energy. Always allow adequate time after a eating a meal for digestion, which during pregnancy is slower than normal. If you have not previously regularly exercised but wish to start some sort of activity during this trimester, then you must first get the approval of your LMC before embarking. Make sure you take it very easy, keeping the intensity gentle and the duration no longer than 20–30 minutes a day.

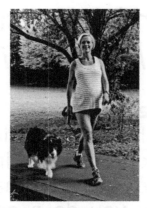

Fig.7.2

✓ **Walking** Walking will increase circulation and may help prevent blood pooling in your lower legs. Arm swinging and a good pace achieved while walking will release the 'feel-good hormones' that accompany aerobic exercise. If the weather is too hot, cold or wet, consider walking on a treadmill. You can do an interval-type walking programme where you vary your pace from fast to slow for a few minutes a time—an active exercise phase followed by a recovery phase.

✗ **Jogging** In reality very few women would consider continuing with this sort of exercise in the third trimester. However, if you do wish to continue jogging during your third trimester, your routine will need to be modified considerably purely for comfort. The weight of your uterus and of the baby pushing down on your already stretched pelvic floor muscles will provide added pressure, so make sure you have emptied your bladder before heading out.

Practise regular pelvic floor lifting, brace your lower abdominals to provide support to your lower back and baby bump, and make sure your warm-up and cool-down are long and slow. Your pace should be no more than a gentle jog, and avoid hills and uneven ground. You may find a pregnancy support belt is also a great help.

✕ **Outdoor cycling** This is not a good choice at this stage, as there is too much risk of a fall or injury with your increased weight and altered centre of gravity. You are far better to choose a stationary cycle, and lift the handle bars up so you are sitting more upright rather than leaning forward.

Home-based and gym cardio equipment

It is personal preference that will determine the sort of equipment you feel most comfortable on. You can always do a cardio workout that utilises several different pieces of equipment; 10–15 minutes on each with short change-over times in between. This will still let you achieve an elevated heart rate but adds variety.

✓ **Stationary bike** During this trimester you must take care in getting on and off the bike seat due to your unstable pelvis and your altered sense of balance. Lift the handlebars up high to avoid bending forward at the hips, and modify intensity according to your perceived rate of exertion.

√ **Elliptical trainer** This machine is fine to continue using. Make sure you warm up slowly with little resistance, because this machine uses both your arms and legs, which means your heart rate will elevate quickly. Consider not using the moveable arm part of the machine if you are finding balancing a challenge. Some machines allow you to disable the arm extensions. You will naturally be leaning forward a little as you use this machine, so make sure you tilt from the hips, and avoid over-arching your lower back by tucking your tailbone under slightly and drawing in your abdominals (draw your baby towards you). Avoid rounding the back or shoulders.

× **Stepper** Only continue to use this machine if you can maintain pelvic alignment when balancing on one leg, so that you are not putting undue strain on your already hormonally weakened pelvic region. Stepping with a big tummy out front can be cumbersome and awkward. It is suitable to use as part of your workout, but not for any extended length of time: use it for 10–15 minutes, and then continue your cardio workout using another machine, such as a recumbent cycle or the treadmill.

× **Rower** Not the most comfortable choice at this point, as it is physically difficult to reach the rowing bar, and repetitively leaning forward puts extra pressure on your abdomen and back as well as potentially compressing your baby.

✓ **Treadmill** A good piece of equipment for beginners as it is adaptable to all fitness levels by adjusting both intensity and gradient. It works the legs and buttocks and is a very functional activity. Bonus: using a treadmill can be done in any sort of weather and can be quite social with a friend using a machine alongside you.

Water-supported exercise

Swimming, aqua jogging, and aqua aerobics are all good to continue during your third trimester. If beginning any of these at this stage, make sure you take it extremely gently and advise the class instructor. It may be a chance each week for you to actually get to feel 'light' again. Enjoy the water buoyancy for the ability it gives you to exercise aerobically, but also for its relaxation effect. A couple of good activities to try are squats in chest-deep or low-level water, or slow-stepping backward lunges in chest-deep water. Both moves strengthen the leg and buttock muscles involved in common birthing positions. If you are more agile, try a jump lunge where you propel your body up in the water and switch your feet front to back. (If you suffer from pubic symphysis or pelvic discomfort, don't do this movement.) Allow some time after exercising to just float, supported on buoyancy aids if you desire. If you are experiencing blood pressure issues at this stage of your pregnancy (typically elevated blood pressure), being in shoulder-deep water can help decrease your overall blood pressure. However, do not do any sort of water exercise if your waters have broken, as it will put you at risk of infection.

√ **Swimming** Swimming during your third trimester is an excellent choice, as the feeling of floating and being weightless provides a welcome relief for tired joints, ligaments and muscles that are working hard to support your increased size. You may find you have to decrease your swimming speed. This activity is one you can do every day if you choose. Another option is to intersperse swimming lengths with aqua jogging or pool walking.

√ **Aqua jogging** This is another good exercise for this stage of pregnancy due to the buoyancy factor. You may find lifting your knees up high is restricted by your baby bump, but you can still get a reasonable stride length. Warm up with some walking lengths first, and do some gentle stretches in the water afterwards using the edge of the pool for support. Other options for exercising in water at this stage are holding on to the edge of the pool and kicking, or using a flutter board for kicking lengths.

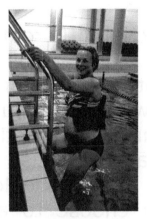
Fig.7.3

✓ **Aqua aerobics** Make sure the instructor knows you are pregnant so they can show you modifications for any moves that might be difficult for you. It is unlikely that you would be doing anything so vigorous that you would cause an injury; however, due to the amount of relaxin in your system by this stage, you need to be aware, even in water, of not flinging your legs around as you may strain your pubic symphysis region. The sort of movement that may exacerbate a problem is sideways travelling squatting moves, which involve the legs stepping apart and then in again with the added pressure of water resistance. Just keep your movements in the frontal plane by turning to face the direction of movement and either walk or lunge instead of squatting. Don't feel you need to complete the entire class or every move, just work within your comfort level.

Group fitness classes

In this section I outline pregnancy modifications for a variety of Les Mills classes as their group fitness programme is available in 80 countries worldwide, but of course they are not the only class options. There are many other suitable exercise classes you can attend at gyms and in the local community. If the class you choose to attend is similar in content to those outlined here then cast your eye over the modifications and adapt as necessary. As a general rule, for *any class* you should always let the instructor know you are pregnant so they can provide additional cueing and offer alternative movements that are more suitable for pregnancy. If you feel the instructor does not have the knowledge to modify the movements accordingly, then use your own sensible judgement and always err on the side of caution. Do less rather than more.

The third trimester is not the time to begin a new activity or group fitness class. However, if you have already been participating throughout your pregnancy in various classes, then some are suitable to continue with provided you proceed with caution; others you may have to bypass. Unless you are attending a class specifically for pregnant women, you will find that many moves will need to be adjusted. It is not possible to list all the sorts of moves you will need to change, but any form of high-impact, bouncing or fast movement will likely be uncomfortable, and you may find that the duration of the class is challenging. Don't lie on your stomach, and avoid extended periods on your back. Try to maintain good posture and low-grade abdominal bracing throughout. Take regular breaks. Walk on the spot, sip water regularly, and perhaps position yourself at the rear of the class so you can take as many 'time outs' as you need without feeling as if you are hindering the class flow. Use all the low-impact options offered to you by the instructor.

~ **Cycle classes** If you wish to continue with cycle classes during your third trimester there are certain modifications that are recommended. When getting on the bike, sit on the seat sideways first and ease around to face forward, minimising the movement of separating your legs to avoid pelvic strain. Reverse this action to dismount.

Raise the handlebars high so that you have a very small tip forward at the hips, if any. Avoid standing up on the pedals for extended periods. Adjust pedal resistance to keep your RPE to around 5. Drink plenty of water. Keep cool by sitting in a well-ventilated area, and wear layers of clothing you can peel off. Consider sitting at the back of the class so you can coast when you need to, and thus not feel any pressure to keep up with the other class participants. Don't feel the need to complete the entire class, do as much as you feel able and then either cool down on a treadmill or with stretches.

~ **Aerobics classes** Discuss your participation in the class with the instructor to make sure they are confident in providing you with plenty of alternative movements suitable for your late stage of pregnancy. In general, as your pregnancy progresses you may decide to minimise or cut out impact, twisting or complex choreography. Stand at the rear of the class so you can march on the spot or take a break whenever you need it. Monitor your heat level, hydration and heart rate carefully, taking care not to overdo it. Make your participation focus 'easy movement and fun' rather than hard effort.

~ **Step classes** Seeing the step beyond your extended belly may be the first challenge you face with this class. Only those who are experienced with step classes should continue with this form of exercise during the third trimester. Modify by just using the step itself at this stage, with no risers. You could even choose to do the moves on the floor with no step at all. Take care with sideways squatting moves or twisting moves.

✕ **Combat/Kick-boxing/Cross-fit-type classes** Not suitable for the third trimester, due to the explosive nature of movements and the potential risk of falls or injury.

✕ **Circuit classes** Generally, circuit classes are not suitable for the third trimester due to the high intensity and speed of movements. The exception would be a specific prenatal class. Discuss with your LMC and the class instructor to make sure there will be suitable alternative moves offered to you and that they are happy for you to take part. Always err on the side of caution, and if an activity doesn't feel right, stop. It may be time to consider another form of exercise, like using a treadmill or swimming.

✓ **BODYBALANCE™** This gentle, low-impact exercise involves breathing, stretching and strengthening, and is suitable, with modification, for the third trimester. If you are new to this class, make sure you tell the instructor you are pregnant, and have the alternative recommended moves for this late stage of pregnancy demonstrated to you prior to the session. Gyms offering BODYBALANCE™ classes should be able to provide you with a specific pregnancy guide for this class that includes photos of the recommended modifications for pregnant participants.

General BODYBALANCE™ Modifications

Advise the instructor that you are pregnant so they can provide appropriate verbal cues. Do not feel you need to do every track or every move. Even though this is a relatively gentle class, there are still moves that require reasonable effort and intensity, so don't be afraid to pull back on the effort you exert by about 30%. It is important to still achieve the correct posture and alignment in the various poses and stretches, but flow through the moves gently rather than forcing them. Work only within your normal range of movement. Due to your altered centre of gravity and baby bump, you need to have an extra-stable base of support, so whenever you are in a standing position, make sure your feet are slightly wider than hip-distance apart. Avoid all jumping moves. Instead, step out one foot at a time and consider replacing lunges with a squat move especially if you have any history of sacroiliac or pubic symphysis discomfort or dysfunction. When bending forward from standing or sitting, keep your legs apart to give your baby bump plenty of room. Avoid positions called 'three-legged dog' and 'standing split'. When in standing positions, tuck your tailbone under and avoiding overarching your lower back. Work at your own pace and take a break whenever you need to: the rest of the class are not pregnant—you are! Comfortable positions to rest in are 'child's pose' or 'seated star pose'. Each class follows a set format, so here are more detailed modifications for the sort of moves and adaptations you can make in each track.

Specific track modifications:

- **Track 2—sun salutations** Yoga basis. Feet hip-width apart. If you don't feel comfortable with moves to the floor, do the standing moves and replace 'crocodile', 'cobra' and 'up dog' poses with 'cat stretch', if desired.

- **Track 4—balance** Due to your shape and changing centre of gravity, balancing is challenging, so consider replacing the balance poses on one leg with having both feet on the ground, or use the wall for extra support.

- **Track 6—core abdominals** Modify the moves to abdominal bracing instead, interspersed with pelvic tilts and a set of pelvic floor squeezes in four-point kneeling. No sit-ups or twisting moves, and limit time on your back even if you have no symptoms of supine hypo-extension syndrome (dizziness, nausea, feeling faint.) If you experience any of these, immediately roll over on to your side, and slowly sit up. The instructor may demonstrate some alternative moves that you can try for this track like 'bridging' or a 'hindi squat'; take care with the latter move if you have any history of pelvic or pubic symphysis pain.

- **Track 7—core back** Modify the lying position to four-point kneeling. Switch on your core muscles and use your lower abdominals to maintain a neutral spine. Use the 'camel' pose instead of the 'bow' pose. Keep your legs strong, your chest lifted, and head and neck relaxed.

● **Track 8—twists** When twisting, turn away from the bent knee and minimise the turn movement so there is no compression of your baby.

● **Track 9—forward bends** Legs apart when bending forward, and don't drop your head below your knees. Modify to a back flat position with bent knees, and support your trunk weight with your elbows resting on your thighs.

● **Track 10—relaxation/meditation** Lie on your side for this relaxing conclusion to the class. Be particularly aware of the 'relaxed deep breathing', as you may find this proves a good coping technique for use in early labour.

The information for pregnancy modifications for Les Mills BODYBALANCE™ has been supplied by Les Mills International and specifically addresses pregnancy modifications recommended for this class (as at 2012).

Strength training

This is not the time to begin doing a BODYPUMP™ class, but if you have been participating throughout your pregnancy in this class, then with modification you should be able to complete most tracks. Gyms providing the Les Mills range of group fitness classes should be able to provide you with a BODYPUMP™ pregnancy guide.

Although the instructor should clearly be able to see you are in an advanced stage of pregnancy, it is worth specifically mentioning it to them so they can give you plenty of cues for movement modifications.

General BODYPUMP™ modifications

As in the second trimester, continue with a wider-than-hip-distance standing stance for stability, but not so wide that it will cause stress on your pelvis. Decrease your weights again from what you were lifting in the second trimester. For some tracks you may only use the bar or small plates. For bench tracks, increase the incline angle again from the second trimester. Keep your movements smooth and controlled. You may find better control by using a shorter range of movement. Maintain good core muscle activation, and be aware of good erect posture in standing with a neutral spine. Avoid leaning back or over-arching your lower back. Take care getting down on to the inclined bench, and move out of lying on the bench by rolling to the side. However, you may find that even lying on an inclined bench now is not comfortable, so try arm exercises in half-kneeling or standing positions. You will need to modify the usual abdominal exercises to focus on deep abdominals.

For any of the exercise options with weights above your head, don't feel an obligation to complete all the repetitions, just work within a comfortable range and remember to breathe evenly. Consider cutting down the actual number of repetitions by doing one repetition to the instructor's two. If you think you may feel self-conscious not keeping up with the class, then choose a position at the rear of the room so you can take regular breaks and work at your own pace.

Specific track modifications

See Figs 6.3 and 6.4 for some position modifications.

● **Track 2—legs/squats** Lower your weights, just a bar is sometimes enough. If you are using a barbell with plates, get someone to lift the bar for you and place it on your shoulders. Squat position is just slightly wider than the shoulders, but not too wide. Draw in and engage your lower abdominals, avoid excessive curve in your lower back. Zip up your pelvic floor. Breathe evenly throughout the exercise. Decrease the range of movement if required.

● **Track 3—chest** Incline the bench for comfort, transition carefully getting down onto it and then for getting off—roll to the side rather than sitting forward and up. If you get dizzy or nauseous, roll to the side and sit up. Try beginner press-ups in four-point kneeling, bending your elbows to lower your chest to the ground.

● **Track 4—back/gluteals/hamstrings** Consider using plates rather than the bar for moves above your head like the 'clean and press'. Don't hold your breath, and if you get any dizziness when using your arms above your head, stop and use an upright row move instead. Keep your wrists strong and slightly extended during the 'clean' phase of the clean-and-press action. Focus on rolling the shoulders back and squeezing your shoulder blades together: this helps maintain strength in your upper back as more load is progressively placed on your spine due to your increasing breast size.

● **Track 5—arms/triceps** Incline the bench for extensions, presses and pullovers. If you prefer to not lie down, then try a seated position for tricep extension work and use a plate instead of the bar. Intersperse this with tricep kickbacks on your hands and knees. Dips off the edge of the bench are fine, but you may need to extend your legs out further to accommodate your baby bump.

● **Track 6—legs/lunges** If you have any history of sacroiliac problems or pelvic instability, use a squat instead of a lunge. Avoid stepping lunges or jumping lunges. Static lunges with a smaller range of movement should be fine, or replace it with a squat option instead. Pay attention to correct body posture by really focusing on keeping your trunk upright without leaning back. Engage and pull in your deep abdominals throughout the exercise to support the lower back.

● **Track 7—abdominals** Do abdominal bracing in four-point kneeling for this track, then do some pelvic tilts, then do as many pelvic floor exercises as you can until the music finishes. You can also do side-lying crunches with a modified range of movement.

The information for pregnancy modifications for Les Mills BODYPUMP™ has been supplied by Les Mills International and specifically addresses pregnancy modifications recommended for this class (as at 2012).

Own strength-training programme

If you have already been participating in strength training, then continue with your exercises, keeping your weights relatively low to just maintain tone and strength. The third trimester of pregnancy is not a time to increase weights or try new exercises unless you are under the guidance of a personal trainer who has specific expertise in training women in a late stage of pregnancy. As you get larger, it is likely you will have to alter your programme as you may not physically be comfortable using and fitting into position on some gym machines. Reduce your weights by a further 5–10% this trimester, so that equates to about a third of what you would have lifted pre-pregnancy. Reduce the number of sets to 2 and aim for 10–20 repetitions. Your effort level now should be only mild to moderate, and you should not be straining hard or 'working to failure'. During this trimester you may benefit from training with someone else so they can be on hand to assist you for your final few repetitions, or to pass weights to you once you are in position. Make sure you continue to breathe evenly throughout your workout, as holding your breath can cause your blood pressure to rise.

Machine or free-weights strength exercises for the third trimester (with modifications)

These are not the only exercises you can do, but they cover the main muscle groups safely and effectively if you are doing your own unsupervised strength workout in a gym setting. If you are unsure of correct technique, get an instructor to demonstrate the exercise for you first.

LOWER BODY

1 Squats with dumbbells

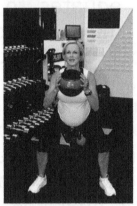

Fig.7.4

Squats with dumbbells or a medicine ball, rather than a barbell, are still a good functional exercise provided you do not have any problems with your back or hips. Wall squats are an alternative (see later description of the technique).

2 Incline leg-press machine

This machine will gradually become difficult to use, because bringing your legs towards your chest will compress your baby. The only exception would be if the movement is of lesser range than normal, so your bent knees do not touch your abdomen. You can adjust some machines to give a smaller range of movement. Supine (lying face up) leg-presses are not suitable at this stage of pregnancy.

3 Lunges

Lunges are also a good functional exercise to do, but if you have pelvis or knee problems avoid them. Avoid stepping lunges, but static lunges are fine. Make sure your legs are shoulder-distance apart before you step one leg forward in order to get a stable base of support. Check your alignment and modify the range of movement if necessary. If you find balancing difficult, consider stabilising yourself with one hand on a wall.

4 Standing hamstring curl

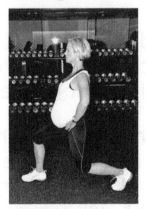

Fig.7.5

Maintain neutral spine as a starting position, and switch on your deep abdominals to brace as you lift your heel up.

5 Seated leg extension

Keep your back pressed into the seat support with shoulders down, and keep breathing evenly throughout.

UPPER BODY

1 Lat pull-down

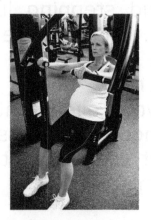

Fig.7.6

Pull the bar down in front of your body to no lower than chin height, concentrating on squeezing your shoulder blades together.

2 Seated horizontal chest-press

This position is quite safe and supportive, so just make sure you maintain good trunk posture throughout, with even breathing.

3 Single-arm cable chest-press

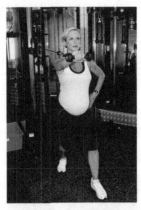

Fig.7.7

Create a stable base with a split-leg stance, keeping hips locked and facing forwards, not twisting as you move. Activate your obliques (side abdominals) and chest muscles to perform a controlled upper body movement, extending your arm forward from the shoulder and returning with a slight upper-body twist.

4 Seated or standing over-head-press

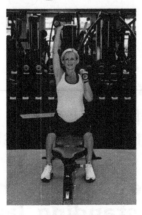

Fig.7.8

This is suitable only if you can maintain good spine alignment. Keep the weights low so that you are not straining, and avoid holding your breath. Consider doing alternate arm lifts rather than bilateral.

5 Seated row with a single- or double-hand pulley

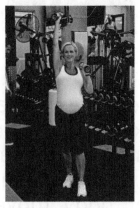

Fig.7.9

Bend your knees slightly or sit to take the strain off your lower back.

ARMS

1 Tricep kickback
One knee supported on a bench, switch on your core to maintain good straight alignment of your spine.
2 Seated bicep curl with dumbbells
3 Seated or standing lateral raise with dumbbells
4 Upright row with dumbbells

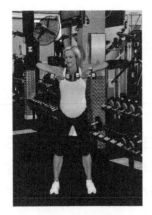

Fig.7.10

ABDOMINALS

Deep abdominal work should continue throughout this trimester to give support to your spine and to your increasingly expanding and heavy baby bump. Hands and knees, side-lying, sitting or standing are the preferred position for exercises to be performed. Towards the latter stage of this trimester the number of abdominal exercises, as well as the length of static holds, can be gradually reduced. Lying on your back is not recommended. If you have symptoms of carpal tunnel syndrome as mentioned previously, then avoid the flexed hand position required for four-point kneeling. You may find great relief for back aches and strain by performing a set of pelvic tilts in any one of the positions listed below. This can offer particular relief at night prior to getting into bed.

1 Brace then tilt

A pelvic tilt describes the action of the lower spine and pelvis tucking under, without necessarily much abdominal activity, but if you add an abdominal brace to a tilt you have an effective safe exercise for this trimester. So in each of the positions below, draw in your lower abdominals and brace your tummy then perform the tilt movement.

A Four-point pelvic tilts

Starting position: Get on all fours, with your hands under your shoulders and your knees under your hips. Keep your elbows and back in a neutral position, and your head in line with your spine.

Action: Draw in and brace your abdominals, then tilt your pelvis under by contracting those deep abdominals. Pull your baby up towards your spine and hold the contraction for 5 seconds, breathe evenly.

B Standing pelvic tilts

Starting position: Stand erect with a good upright posture, shoulders down and back, with pelvis in neutral. Your feet should be shoulder-width apart, and your knees slightly bent.

Action: Draw in and brace your abdominals, then tilt your pelvis so that your tailbone tucks under. Draw in and brace your abdominals as you do so. Hold this position for 5 seconds, then gently release to neutral. Repeat 10 times.

C Wall-supported pelvic tilts

Starting position: Stand with your back against a wall, your feet shoulder-width apart and your heels about 30 centimetres from the wall, with knees slightly bent.

Action: Draw in and brace your abdominals, then tilt your pelvis until your lower back flattens against the wall. Draw in and brace your abdominals as you perform the movement. Hold this position for 5 seconds. Repeat 10 times.

D Side-lying pelvic tilts

Starting position: Lying on your side.

Action: Draw in and brace your abdominals then tuck your tailbone under. Complete a set of 10.

2 Side-lying hip-hitching

Starting position: Lie on your side with your top leg straight and bottom leg bent. Your head can rest on your outstretched bottom arm in a comfortable position, or you can use a small pillow as support.

Action: Draw in and brace your abdominals, then raise your top leg about 5 centimetres and hold it in this position. Next, use your side abdominal muscles to pull your hip toward your shoulder, keeping the top leg straight as you

368

pull. Hold 5 seconds and repeat 10 times. Note: Your bottom leg should not move during this exercise.

Dear Diary—Beach bliss

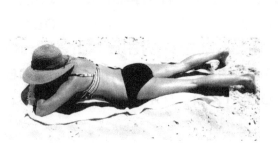

Fig.7.11

A trip to the beach today necessitated a hole being dug in the sand to house my baby bump. It's the first time I've been able to lie on my tummy for months—bliss! I had my 31-week check today and baby is on track to be fairly big, charting above the upper percentile line for growth. The main news was that baby is now head-down feet-up, which is great. It is an ideal position to be in at this stage, and generally they don't revert once they've made the move to this position. It certainly accounts for the massive amount of alien-like rolling and acrobatics I've been feeling in recent days.

Flexibility

The pregnancy hormone relaxin is working its magic on all the ligaments and tendons in your body by softening them in preparation for the expansion required during the birth process, so during the third trimester you must not overstretch or extend your body further than your normal range of movement. Overstretching could lead to injury or joint instability that can last well beyond pregnancy. Your joints also have less synovial fluid in them, meaning less cushioning, which makes you more prone to injury from jolting or jarring. Some days all you will feel like doing is a few stretches—at these times, remember the Bare Essentials routine outlined in Appendix A.

Stretch technique

It is important to hold each stretch for the usual 20–30 seconds, but avoid temptation to press further into the position, even if you suddenly feel a whole lot more flexible. Get yourself into comfortable supported positions for each stretch and concentrate on your breathing. Use your stretch time as a chance to focus on relaxation of body and mind—making your breaths slower and deeper. This is your treat time for exercising.

Stretches for the third trimester

Refer back to the stretch photos (Fig.6.17). Where an exercise is marked *, this indicates that it is particularly important, as these muscles get tight towards the latter stages of pregnancy.

With ball

√ Hip flexor stretch with one hand on ball*

√ Double-arm pull-back off the ball

√ Sitting side-stretch on the ball

√ Hamstrings—sitting on the ball, bend from hips, ankles flexed, one leg extended at a time*

√ Chest and shoulder single-arm diagonals pull-back

√ Sitting spine swivel, rotating the upper body around and looking behind

Standing

√ Doorway chest-opener, alternate arm, the 'stop' position*

√ Calf stretch – straight- and bent-knee

√ Standing quads stretch—one hand on wall

Sitting

Avoid sitting with your legs wide apart if you have back or pelvic pain, and take care getting down on to and up off the floor.

√ Cat stretch—on hands and knees, arch your back up, pelvis tucked under

√ Sitting butterfly adductor stretch

√ Standing with chair abductor stretch—hold on to the chair for balance, and lift one leg onto the seat of the chair, then bend the supporting leg and maintain an abdominal brace as you lean forward

√ Side-lying quads stretch

Pilates

If you have already been attending Pilates classes throughout your pregnancy, then you should have no problems continuing on during the third trimester for as long as you feel able, although if you haven't already switched to a specific prenatal Pilates session now is a good time to do so. One-on-one sessions with an instructor are also an option, and consider shorter length sessions of 30 minutes rather than a full hour. The balance of flexibility and strengthening with reinforcement of regular pelvic floor and deep abdominal activation will be particularly useful to you during this time, as well as giving you a head-start for resuming gentle exercise after birth.

The instructor should be able to give you appropriate modifications to the various moves or suggest alternative moves. Due to the chance of experiencing symptoms of supine hypotensive syndrome, limit the amount of time you spend lying on your back to just a few minutes or less. Avoid wide leg positions to limit stress on your lower back and pelvis, and limit the amount of time a position or contraction is held. Also ensure you are not holding your breath. Decrease the intensity of effort you put into stretching moves, making sure you only stretch within your normal range of flexibility and not beyond. Take care when moving from one position to another.

Don't feel the need to complete an entire class, just do what feels comfortable for you on any given day.

Yoga

Yoga during this trimester will need to accommodate your growing big belly while preventing any compression of your baby. While it is common for your energy levels to progressively diminish, yoga is an activity you may be comfortable continuing right up until term, as you can adjust the intensity depending on how you feel. Your new shape is an important consideration in the poses you do, as well as getting down on to and up from the floor.

Mainstream yoga classes will require extensive modification as there are poses that are not recommended for this advanced stage of pregnancy, so it is best to attend a prenatal yoga session with an experienced instructor who has knowledge of advising pregnant participants.

Remember you are in control of what you do, and if at any stage you don't feel comfortable performing a pose then skip it. Put into practice one of the skills that yoga encourages, and listen to your body. Yoga incorporates valuable breathing and mental relaxation techniques which can be helpful in calming the mind and alleviating any anxieties you may feel about the impending birth process or other stresses in your life. Pay particular attention to mastering the breath with long inhalations through the nose and exhalations through the mouth, as an ability to calm and centre yourself through such a breathing technique can come in handy during labour. Some women comment on how practising yoga gives them an increased sense of bonding with their baby. Make sure that the clothing you wear is loose enough to allow you to move freely but not so flowing as that it will get in the way.

General modifications

● The usual cautions for stretching while pregnant apply – only work within your usual range of movement, do not be tempted or encouraged to push further or deeper into stretches, as due to your increased joint and ligament laxity (due to pregnancy hormones) you could injure yourself. Stretch and hold positions only to the point of mild tension, not pain, and as your pregnancy progresses decrease the length of time you hold a particular pose, around 10–20 seconds is adequate. Be particularly careful of your knee joints.

● Yoga positions have a definite focus on good posture, but in particular be aware of drawing in and bracing your abdominals, zipping up your pelvic floor muscles, and achieving alignment of a neutral spine by tucking your tailbone under slightly to avoid over-arching your lower back.

● Avoid poses that require you to lie for an extended period on your back, due to the risk of supine hypotensive syndrome.

● Make space for your baby bump when bending forwards by taking a slightly wider stance to avoid any compression. If you have hip, back or pubic symphysis problems, avoid taking your legs too far apart when either standing or sitting. Any twisting should be attempted with care and within a short range of movement, try turning more from your shoulders than your hips. An open twist position may be more suitable, which means twisting away from your forward leg.

● Modify any balance moves, and use either the wall or a chair for added support.

● Obviously lying on your tummy is out. Avoid jumping into or out of poses, as well as any rapid breathing or breath-holding, abdominal work, back bends and inversions.

● Avoid Bikram (hot yoga), and certain forms of yoga that involve dynamic moves may be too intense for this stage of pregnancy.

● This is not the time to overdo it. If in doubt, leave it out.

Relaxation

Relaxation = the refreshment of body or mind. Relaxation of both the mind and the body are equally important and beneficial. It goes without saying that a prolonged level of stress during pregnancy is not good for either you or the baby's wellbeing. Elevated mental stress often exhibits itself through physical symptoms, such as tight muscles, headaches, insomnia, fatigue, digestive disorders, and blood pressure problems.

In extreme cases, high stress can cause disturbances to your circulation and digestion, which can impact the growth of the baby. We live in a world where stress and stressful situations are an everyday occurrence. The demands on our time and the speed at which we travel through life all account for a certain amount of stress. In a non-pregnant state most of us ride the typical roller-coaster of positive and negative stress, and in an ideal world take time out when the latter is high in order to dissipate it. During this third trimester rest and relaxation are just as important as exercise.

There are many factors that may result in increased levels of mental tension and stress for you during this time. Of course there are the usual culprits like work, financial or relationship pressures. But you may also have extra stressors, such as concerns about the actual labour, the addition of a new family member, the responsibility of looking after a newborn and even redefining how you see yourself. Add to the mix the fact that your hormones are fluctuating, there are multiple demands on your physical body, your usual sleep pattern may be altered, the understandable trepidation about the impending and usually unpredictable birth process, and it is clear to see pregnant women have every reason to be a little tense! Recognising rising stress and managing it is the key to ensuring an enjoyable journey through these last few months of your pregnancy.

The mind

Relaxation of the mind involves quietening the 'chatty monkey' that exists between your ears. One way is by using a focusing technique whereby you eliminate random thoughts by concentrating hard on perhaps a word, a sound, or an image. Practice is the key to success. Meditation techniques are a great tool for ridding your mind of unnecessary chatter, and you may wish to investigate these further. Other simple ways of dealing with mental stress are talking about any issues with someone or writing down your concerns. These are ways of unloading the burden. While you may not find an immediate solution, there is a saying that often rings true: 'a problem shared is a problem halved'. Talking to other pregnant women or other mothers of a similar age can be incredibly valuable, both in terms of alleviating concerns and providing reassurance that you can and will cope with the changing circumstances. Dumping down all your worries on paper, even down to the tiniest niggle can really help you de-stress. You may even need the listening ear and objective perspective of a counsellor. If you find your levels of stress and anxiety are high and sustained, please discuss the matter with your LMC. They have your mental and physical wellbeing foremost, and will no doubt be able to provide you with suggestions of how you can best relieve any tension. It may even be a simple case of some pregnancy-related issue requiring further explanation.

You may have already enrolled and be attending antenatal classes, which discuss and educate new mothers on many elements that may be causing concern. Many classes also involve a tour of the facility where you plan to give birth; if not, this can usually be coordinated through your LMC. It is well worth the effort to visit the hospital or birthing unit, as familiarising yourself with its location, staff, and the birthing options you may be offered will make you feel more in control, even though the birth process is largely an unpredictable journey.

The body

One of the best ways to unwind tight muscles and a tense physical body is by mastering 'the breath', making it deeper, slower and under your control. It is often said that the breath is the bridge between body and mind. Learning to breathe better is one of the most basic and effective forms of relaxing. Conscious control of your breathing can slow it down, make it deeper and help unwind your body and mind. Tension and stress tend to make the breath shorter and shallower, which is often referred to as 'chest breathing'. Chest breathing provides us with the least amount of oxygen and tightens the surrounding neck and shoulder muscles. In fact, if you get really tight in your neck and shoulders, it could well be a symptom of persistent shallow breathing.

The kind of breathing to master is belly breathing (diaphragmatic breathing). This means deep, long, slow, open, relaxed breaths; the sort of breathing required of opera singers. Diaphragmatic breathing encourages maximum oxygen intake, which in turn helps reduce muscle tension. An awareness and ability to switch to effective belly breathing is both an excellent relaxation technique and a useful tool during early labour.

Take a moment now to notice where you are breathing. Put one hand on your chest and the other below your ribs. Is your breathing more up or down? Is it even? Is it deep or shallow? In the few moments you have taken to analyse your breathing, you will have slowed it down and started to breathe deeper.

Belly breathing: how it's done

Begin in a supported half-lying position; once you have learnt the technique, you will be able to do it standing, sitting, anywhere, any time. Place one hand below your ribs, in the centre of your abdomen. Take a long, deep breath, slowly and calmly, fill your lungs with air, and feel your abdomen swelling as you do so. The air travels through your nose, down your wind pipe, and down in to the lowest chambers of your lungs. Imagine the passage of the air. Take in normal-sized breaths and you should feel your stomach swell out slightly, making your hand rise. As you exhale, your abdomen sinks back in. Don't force it—just relax and let it flow! Put your other hand high on your chest to check that the movement there is minimal. Ninety per cent of the action should be happening lower down, not in the upper chest area. Focus on your exhalation, sighing the breath out and releasing and relaxing as you do so. Let go physically and mentally. Now rest your hands by your sides and carry on doing relaxed belly breathing for at least 10 slow breaths. Notice the difference in your body tension and stress levels. Even focusing on something as simple as breathing for a few minutes can help you unwind. Good times to practise belly breathing are at the end of your exercise sessions during your stretches, in bed at night to help calm your mind prior to sleep, or anytime you feel yourself becoming stressed. Pause, take a moment to belly breathe, and flush away the tension.

Massage

Many women find a specific pregnancy massage a wonderful form of relaxation. Massage can be done at any point during pregnancy, but make sure you seek out a qualified practitioner who specialises in massaging pregnant women, as there are certain techniques and areas of your body that are best avoided during this time. Word of mouth is often the best recommendation; your LMC may also be able to refer you to someone suitable. In order to be massaged effectively and safely during this time, you will either be positioned on your side with plenty of pillows to support you, or there may be a special table that has a gap for your baby bump. Lying on your back is not recommended for any length of time at this late stage of pregnancy.

Exercise itself

Exercising has always been a great way of dealing with mental and physical tension. During this trimester if you are able to include gentle to moderate regular exercise sessions it will help you manage stress buildups. If the pressures of work or running a busy house mean you are unable to achieve your planned workout, then running through a few stretches will enhance both mental and physical relaxation. Consider the 15-minute Bare Essentials routine in Appendix A.

Dear Diary—30 weeks and counting

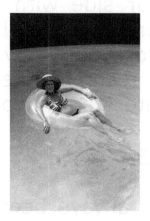

Fig.7.12

I am currently staying at a hotel that has a lap swimming pool with chest-depth water, so I went 'running' in it today. No floatation device needed. I just literally ran up and down the pool, arms under the water pumping back and forth. When I got bored I swam a few laps to break it up. It wasn't too energetic, but enough to make me feel revitalised. In fact at present 30–40 minutes total for a workout is plenty for me. I am also finding that when I wake up I'm not bouncing out of bed ready for the day. Maybe it's due to the fact that I'm getting broken sleep because of getting up and down to pee, plus all the manoeuvring in bed with a pillow between my knees. Or maybe it's because I'm no spring chicken any more. However, if I urge myself to do just a little exercise early in the day then the pay-off is great. I generally feel quite vital afterwards and for the next few hours. I also have noticed I might need a little nana-nap in the afternoon, which again is completely normal for this stage; top-up sleeps should be encouraged!

Two home workouts

Both of these workouts are designed to take 40 minutes maximum. The first is a toning and stretching workout to be done at home, and covers all the main muscle groups; the second is a walking routine with relevant stretches included.

What you will need

Space

An area to work out in of about 2 metres square. If it's fine weather you might want to consider doing some of the exercises outside.

Equipment

A towel or a mat. A Swiss ball, and a stretchy band or flex band/tube to provide resistance.

Workout 1: Toning at home

With each exercise: remember to zip up your pelvic floor muscles and brace your abdominals to provide good lower back support and strong core stabilisation throughout.

Beginner level: 1 set of each exercise (after a few sessions you can increase to 2 sets).

Previously active and fit prior to pregnancy: 2 sets, completing each exercise in a slow and controlled manner so you feel the exertion but not exhaustion.

1 Wall squats

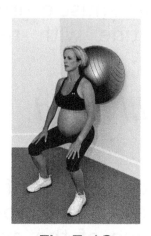

Fig.7.13

This time you can do them leaning into a Swiss ball against the wall. They can also be performed free-standing. See the instructions for 'smooth squats' given in the second trimester home workout.

Muscles used: front and back of thigh, butt and back.

Key points: Your feet should be shoulder-distance apart, with toes slightly turned out. Now walk both feet forward one step so that instead of standing vertically you are leaning into the ball which is against the wall for support. Start with the ball in the centre of your back so that as you squat down it will ride up to your shoulder level. Exhale and take about 2 seconds to squat down, keeping your thighs to 90° or above, no lower. Make sure your knees are tracking out over your toes, not rolling inwards. Hold the squat position for 8–10 seconds, then rise up again and repeat 10 times. You should feel your thighs working hard to hold you steady in the lowered squat position.

1 set: 10 repetitions. Rhythm is 2 seconds, hold 10 seconds, rise up.

A Quads stretch (see Fig.6.17)

Now put your hand against the wall for support and stretch the front of your thigh. Drop the hip of the leg you have lifted down, so that both hip bones are even and facing forward, and your knees are in line.

2 Lunges

Lunges are a very functional activity. For this trimester you can modify the lunge move by how low you choose to go.

Muscles used: legs, butt, back, core.

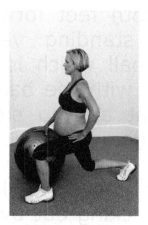

Fig.7.14

Key points: Using the Swiss ball for support, place your hand on the top of the ball, take a wide split-leg stance with an erect upper-body posture, tucking your tailbone under and drawing in your abdominals. Now, lower your back knee towards the floor. You can take the other arm out to the side for stability or place it on your hip. Keep your shoulders back, and the movement smooth and controlled. Remember when you lower down to the floor by bending the knee, there should not be any forward movement at the knee joint.

1 set: 15 each leg. Rhythm is 2 seconds down, 2 seconds up.

***Alternative exercise:* Side-lying leg lifts (abduction)**

If due to knee problems you are unable to perform lunges, then replace with this exercise.

1 set: 20 repetitions each side. Rhythm is 2 seconds up, 2 seconds hold, 2 seconds down.

B Hip flexor stretch (see Fig.6.17)

Using the ball again for support, take one foot forward into a half-kneeling position. Have the ball on the side opposite to the leg that is forward. Place a towel or mat under your bent knee if you are on a hard surface.

3 Donkey kicks

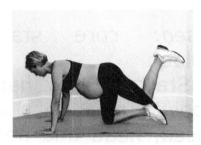

Fig.7.15

Muscles used: butt, back, core.

Key points: On your hands and knees (or resting on your forearms if you have carpal tunnel problems), draw in your abdominals and brace, keeping your back in a neutral position, and your head in line with your spine. Lift one leg with bent knee, and push your heel towards the ceiling, lifting so your thigh is level with your back.

1 set: 20 repetitions each side. Rhythm is 2 seconds up, 2 seconds hold, 2 seconds down.

4 4-point alternate arm lifts

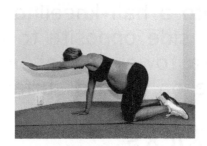

Fig.7.16

Muscles used: core stabilisers, back extensors, shoulder.

Key points: Start on your hands and knees in the four-point position, spine neutral, abdominals braced, head and neck in line with the spine, pelvic floor zipped up. Lift one arm with a bent elbow out to the side horizontally, and slide your hand forward to full arm extension, then reverse the movement. As you lift the arm, squeeze the shoulder blade towards the spine. Keep your hips parallel to the floor and maintain a strong core so you don't sag in the mid-region. Keep the movement slow and controlled.

1 set: 10 each side. Rhythm is 1 second for each phase, up, extend, retract, lower.

C Child's pose stretch

Kneel on floor, separating your knees. Place your big toes together and sit your buttocks back on your heels. Extend your arms above your head on the floor. Pull back and find a comfortable position with your belly between your thighs and upper body relaxed. Keep your head and neck in line with your spine, or rest your forehead on the floor.

5 Lateral raise with flex band

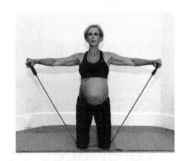

Fig.7.17

Muscles used: core, deltoids.

Key points: Anchor the flex band under both knees, using a towel for padding if you are on a hard surface. Drop your shoulders down and extend and raise the arms either side of your body; the higher you go, the harder the resistance. Keep a slight bend in your elbows throughout, and keep good neutral upper-body posture, not leaning forwards or back.

1 set: 10. Rhythm is 2 seconds up, pause briefly, 2 seconds lower.

6 Kneeling abdominal curl

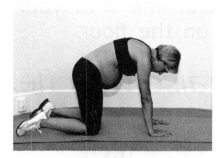

Fig.7.18

This exercise combines a pelvic tilt with abdominal bracing.

Muscles used: core, deep abdominals.

Key points: Kneel in a four-point kneeling position. Draw your abdominals in towards your spine and tuck your tailbone under, rounding your lower back.

1 set: 10. Rhythm is 2 seconds to curl, hold for 5 seconds, release for 2 seconds.

7 Circle mobilisers—hips, arms, ankles and wrists

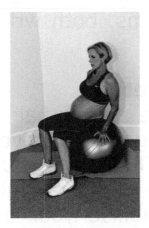

Fig.7.19

Muscles used: core stabilisers, shoulder girdle.

Key points: Sitting comfortably on top of the Swiss ball, feet apart and flat on the floor, begin to rotate your hips so that you are completing a full 360° circle, keeping the movement small to medium in range. Come back to the starting position and complete a set in the reverse direction. This is great mobilisation for your lumbar spine and pelvis.

Arms: One arm at a time, do 10 single backwards full arm rotations with a bent elbow.

Wrists: Rotate both wrists around in one direction for 10 complete circles, then reverse the direction and repeat.

Ankles: One leg at a time, rotate the ankle clockwise 10 times, then anticlockwise 10 times.

1 set: 10 rotations in each direction, for hips, alternate arms, both wrists, and alternate ankles.

D Hamstring stretch

Sitting on the Swiss ball with legs apart, straighten one leg and flex your foot. Now tilt forward from the hips until you feel the muscles on the underside of your thigh stretching. Use your arms to stabilise your body on the bent leg. Hold for 10–15 seconds and repeat on the opposite side.

8 Leg extension on the ball

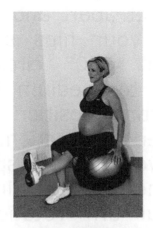

Fig.7.20

Muscles used: core, quadriceps.

Key points: Sitting on the ball, extend one lower leg out to horizontal, then hinge at the knee and bring the heel back to touch the ball. Repeat these leg extensions in a smooth and controlled manner. Switch on your core muscles to keep stable on the ball, but you can use your hands to stabilise either side on the ball if you are wobbling.

1 set: 20 repetitions on each, hold on the 20th repetition for a few seconds, then lower.

9 Wall press-ups

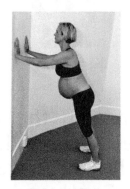

Fig.7.21

Avoid this exercise if you have carpal tunnel problems.

Muscles used: chest, core stabilisers.

Key points: Stand about a metre away from the wall with your hands slightly lower than shoulder level, but wider than shoulder-distance apart. Tuck your tailbone under and brace your abdominals. Bend your elbows and lower your chest to almost touch the wall while maintaining a straight body-line, then reverse the move, pressing through the heels of your hands and

394

squeezing your chest muscles to take you back to the starting position.

1 set: 10–15. Rhythm is slow and controlled: 2 seconds in, 2 seconds out.

E Doorway chest-opener

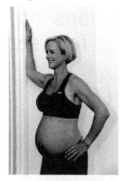

Fig.7.22

To open and stretch the chest, stand in a doorway with one arm in the 'stop' position, forearm against the door frame, body facing through the door. Gently advance through the doorway until you feel a stretch in the chest. Repeat on the other side.

F Spine and neck stretch

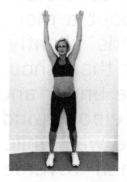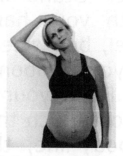

Fig.7.23

Spine: Standing with your back against a wall, heels slightly out from the wall, raise your arms up over your head and stretch your fingers up to the ceiling, keeping your back pressed against the wall to maintain neutral spine. Hold for 10 seconds, keep breathing, lower and repeat.

Neck: Drop your ear directly down towards your shoulder. You can apply a little extra pressure by placing the hand on the upper side of your head. Hold for 10 seconds each side.

Congratulations, you're done! Drink a big glass of water.

Workout 2: Walk and stretch

This is a stop-start workout that you can tailor to your own fitness level. Rather than going for one longer walk, it is split into two segments with stretches interspersed so that you cover all the main muscles groups, and in particular the areas of the body that often get tight in this stage of pregnancy.

Those with a low level of fitness (whether due to pregnancy complications or past inactivity) should aim for 2x10-minute segments; those women who have exercised throughout their pregnancy and have no complications should aim for 15–20 minutes per segment. The stretches are for everyone no matter what your fitness level. Your effort level when walking should be around 4–5 RPE (rate of perceived exertion) or 'light' to 'somewhat hard'. If you are walking with someone, you should be able to carry on a conversation with them. If you are so out of breath that you cannot chat, then slow down. Swing your arms and be aware of maintaining good posture by tucking your tailbone slightly under while keeping your lower abdominals drawn in, to provide extra support to your back and pelvis due to the weight of your now substantial baby bump. Remember to empty your bladder before you set out, and don't forget to take a water-bottle with you so you can take sips regularly.

Workout outline

Walk 15 minutes
Then find a suitable place to perform a few stretches—a park, beach, or grassy area would be ideal. If your walking route takes you to a more urban environment, then pick out an area to perform the stretches away from busy traffic or pedestrian zones so you don't feel self-conscious.

Stretch break: Fig 7.24

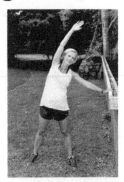

Side stretch

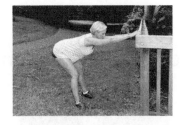

Upper-body pull-back

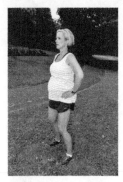

Pelvic tilts—x 10

After completing the stretches above, this is probably your turnaround point so now head back home.

Walk 15 minutes: Fig.7.25

Once home, complete the following stretches.

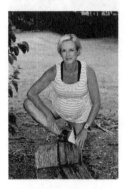

Butt stretch (optional, as it requires you to find something of suitable height to place your leg on)

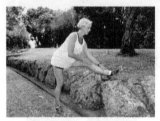

Hamstring

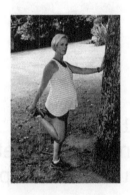

Quads stretch

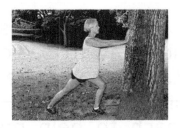

Calf stretch

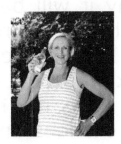

Congratulations you're done! Drink a big glass of water.

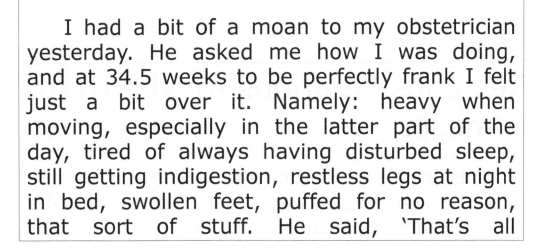

Dear Diary—Fed up

I had a bit of a moan to my obstetrician yesterday. He asked me how I was doing, and at 34.5 weeks to be perfectly frank I felt just a bit over it. Namely: heavy when moving, especially in the latter part of the day, tired of always having disturbed sleep, still getting indigestion, restless legs at night in bed, swollen feet, puffed for no reason, that sort of stuff. He said, 'That's all normal—typical third trimester symptoms', and told me in a nice way to basically suck it up and deal with it. What's that saying? Oh yeah: 'Have a cup of concrete and harden up!' I think the approach to help me manage this fed-up feeling is to rationalise and tell myself this is not the way it will be forever, there is a reason for it all, and there is definitely an endpoint coming. It's also good to consciously switch your thinking from 'ouch that hurts' and 'poor me', to 'isn't my body amazing for coping with these changes and isn't pregnancy incredible'. In other words: reframe it. I know with at least four weeks to go it isn't going to get any easier, so I just need to take a big breath and get on with celebrating the good bits and minimising the uncomfortable bits. I have to say, though, a little bit of empathy from your partner does go a long way. A bit of positive reinforcement that you are doing well all things considered can give a real boost.

Key considerations for the third trimester

This trimester is the growing phase for your baby, which means you get bigger, heavier, and potentially more tired. You may or may not find you suffer from any of the pregnancy complications described earlier in this chapter, but, regardless of whether you are fighting fit or coping with compromise, exercise this trimester is worth doing within your levels of comfort and in consultation with your LMC. Important points to remember are nutrition, hydration and relaxation, so let's recap each one now.

Nutrition

Make sure you are eating a good, healthy, balanced diet. If you find you are suffering from digestion problems, keep your food intake smaller and more frequent. Fuel up before your workout with a small carbohydrate-based snack 30–60 minutes prior. Similarly, you may need to have a small snack after your workout to ensure your blood sugar levels don't drop.

Hydration

Even though you will be visiting the toilet more often this trimester, make sure you keep your fluid intake plentiful, sipping water regularly, especially during and after exercising.

Relaxation

As you progress through this trimester you will need to negotiate a balance of exercise and rest; one shouldn't short-change the other as they are both important. Small periods of rest and relaxation (if that is all you can manage) are better than nothing, and they will go a long way to making your pregnancy journey more enjoyable while keeping you calm in mind and body.

What's the ideal exercise regime?

Use common sense, and if something doesn't feel right, stop doing it. Communicate fully and openly with your LMC; after all, they have your and your baby's best interests at heart. Seek help and advice if you are suffering any of the pregnancy complications mentioned in this chapter, modify your exercise plan accordingly.

Regarding the actual exercise regime, there is no right and wrong or absolute ideal—aside from the general principles of keeping all exercise *moderate* in nature and *regular* if possible. It's all down to how you feel, day to day, week to week, and now is the stage of your pregnancy when you not only must listen to your body but you must give it plenty of tender loving care.

Some women continue with moderate exercise sessions most days of the week, with no adverse effects, right up until giving birth; others will feel they need to taper off both the intensity and duration of their workouts as this trimester progresses. Communicate your exercise intentions to your LMC and heed their advice as regards the overall management of your and your baby's wellbeing. Doing something is better than nothing, but only if it is not causing any exacerbation of symptoms and you feel good doing it. If pregnancy complications mean you are unable to continue with your existing programme, then, with the blessing of your LMC, consider doing the Bare Essentials routine outlined in Appendix A.

Some rest every day is essential in the latter stages of pregnancy. From about 34 weeks on, aim to get a horizontal lie-down every day if possible. You might only be able to achieve 20–30 minutes, even though an hour is ideal, but some rest is better than no rest. Practise belly breathing for relaxation—it is cheap, simple once you know how, can be done anywhere anytime, and is particularly helpful during the early stages of labour to help with pain management.

The weekly plan below is intended as a guide only, as during this trimester it can be just as important to rest if you are feeling fatigued as it is to do some exercise. Above all, keep your exercise sessions fun, simple and low-stress.

Suggested weekly plan

Monday Walk and stretch workout as above, 30 minutes, plus pelvic floor exercises.

Tuesday Aqua jogging, 30 minutes.

Wednesday Day off, or Bare Essentials routine.

Thursday Modified group fitness class.

Friday Walk 20–30 minutes, then do exercises 1, 4, 6 and 7 from the home toning workout.

Saturday Swimming or aqua aerobics class, 30–45 minutes.

Sunday Home toning workout, as above (do as much as you are able), or day off.

Key points

○ Modify, modify, modify.

○ Exercise for fun and for maintenance of your current level of fitness and strength.

○ Gradually tapering off is fine, as is continuing with regular moderate exercise if you are feeling great and your baby is growing healthily.

○ Although your sense of balance may be altered due to your growing belly, the one thing you *can* balance is sufficient exercise as well as rest.

√ Exercise caution during this trimester.
√ Use common sense, if it doesn't feel right—stop.
√ Balance rest and exercise.
√ Practise belly breathing for relaxation.
√ Look forward to the changes ahead.

Dear Diary—The end is in sight

There is one thing that is inevitable now: there's a baby coming out sometime soon. It's weird not knowing when. I'm now 37 weeks or in my 38th week. Baby is above the top percentile of growth for this stage, which is about 3.5 kilos, packing on about 200 grams a week which is much bigger than my first baby at this stage, but that evidently is normal. The obstetrician's scans have a margin of error of 10%-ish, so you can't take the measurements as definitive, but the bump certainly feels heavier and more uncomfortable. I had one day of intense calf pain with no obvious cause, so I spent about seven hours in the Women's Assessment Unit at hospital until they could schedule me for an ultrasound scan of my leg veins to eliminate the possibility of a clot. Pregnancy does make you more predisposed to clots, and if they dislodge and travel elsewhere in the body they can be very serious (fatal), hence the reason I needed the medical all-clear. The scan didn't show anything resembling a clot, and the following day the pain subsided. So I have to put it down to just 'one of those unexplained late-stage pregnancy pains'. I'm also having afternoon naps as necessary. I feel pretty buoyant in the mornings, but then gravity kicks in and I feel as if I have a set of diving weights attached to the bump as the day goes on.

I'm kind of nervous and excited at the same time about what's about to happen. Even though I've been through it once, you can never predict what the second time will be like, except the obstetrician says it's bound to be quicker. Now considering the first was about 4.5 hours that means I can't muck around getting to the hospital, so I'm on alert for the first sign of contractions. Exercise-wise it's a case of as and when possible. The Bare Essentials workout is achievable, but pounding the pavements is out for me now, especially with the summer heat. My body is telling me that rest, pacing myself and getting a decent amount of sleep are the most important things, so that when the birth process does start I have some resilience up my sleeve.

I'm signing off now. It's likely I'll have a new baby when I next do a diary entry ... fingers crossed.

Chapter 8

Bring Back My Body

'The secret to getting ahead is getting started.'
Mark Twain

First, congratulations on your new baby—you made it! Now let me be completely frank and acknowledge that these next few weeks and months are definitely going to be very tiring as you get to grips with your new addition to the family. Although each new mother's journey is specific to her particular circumstances, her baby and her personality, there is a definite common theme of weariness. Whether it is in consistent waves or you reach a point of overwhelming exhaustion (for me this occurred at about six weeks), there is no doubt that caring for a newborn tends to be a mostly relentless routine punctuated by occasional delightful moments. It's amazing in the first few months how much you will be fixated on getting up a burp or two! So, I hear you ask, what on earth is expected of you in terms of exercise and getting back to fitness? Well, not much initially, aside from a few 'non-negotiables' for your own safety and wellbeing.

I have written this chapter in a chronological fashion so you can just read enough for the timeframe you are in. It's split into Phase 1 (0–2 weeks), Phase 2 (2–6 weeks), Phase 3 (6–12 weeks) and Phase 4 (12+ weeks). Time is of the essence with a newborn, and in fact you may find it quite challenging to get *any* time for yourself. So let's be realistic. It took you nine months to grow this gorgeous new baby, so give yourself at least three to nine months to get back to your pre-pregnancy fitness and shape. I am loathe to put timeframes on achieving physical fitness goals at this stage in your life, as the last thing a new mum needs is any sense of failure or pressure. What I can assure you is that if immediately post-birth you follow the non-negotiables and then do the recommended exercises through Phases 2–4, as outlined in this chapter, you *will* recover more quickly and will safely return to being fit and healthy as quickly as possible.

Key points

○ Approaching exercise in bursts of 'little and often' can really work post-birth.

○ Exercising does not affect the quality or quantity of your breast milk.

○ The primary focus for the first 12 weeks is recovery and rejuvenation of weakened and stretched muscles (namely your pelvic floor, abdominals and back), as well as laying the foundations for getting back your pre-pregnancy body.

Caesarean section

If you've had a caesarean birth you're in good company. You probably knew that your chances of having one were increased due to age-related pregnancy complications like:

* high blood pressure
* gestational diabetes
* slow dilation (widening) of the cervix
* having a large baby
* the baby adopting an awkward position in the womb, such as the breech position
* placenta praevia.

If this has been your journey, remember that the first six weeks after having a C-section are the healing phase, and as such your resumption of exercising needs to be further modified compared with if you had a vaginal delivery. You have had a procedure that is classed as major abdominal surgery. You have an abdominal wound that needs to heal without being put under stress. You have also had an epidural, which may result in fluid retention for approximately one week post-delivery, and possibly a sore back where the needle was inserted. Don't push yourself. Don't do any strenuous exercise or heavy lifting for the first couple of months. In fact, for the first six weeks you shouldn't lift anything heavier than your baby. Split baskets of washing into smaller loads. You may wish to wait until after your postnatal check (six weeks) before you attempt any other exercises aside from the non-negotiables and gentle short walks. Check with your LMC or doctor if you wish to resume any further exercising before then.

What you *can* do without any cause for concern is pelvic floor exercises from day one, and deep abdominal bracing from about week two. Then you can slowly add in other exercises from Phase 2 as you feel able. (Note that while Phase 2 covers 2–6 weeks postnatal, for you the timeframe may become closer to 6–10 weeks, and so on for Phases 3 and 4.)

As a general guide, once your wound has healed (the gentle lower tummy exercises will actually help healing and keep the scar region flexible) and you have succeeded in activating your deep abdominal bracing, then you can resume with the Phase 2 programme as normal and continue your progression from there. If you have had any delayed healing of your wound due to infection, check with your LMC or doctor before resuming exercise.

Dear Diary—Week 1

I'm glad to be home with our new baby ... I really am, but I feel totally bashed and bruised. I remember coming home with our first-born and feeling fearful that I was now all on my own looking after this little bundle. This time, with number two, there's a sense of comfort in knowing I have done it before and lived to tell the tale. I know these first few weeks are going to be hard work and exhausting, but I'm still feeling euphoric that we have a healthy baby. I have aches and twinges occurring in random places all over my body. The middle of my back aches; I wonder if that's from the epidural? I must be very careful with lifting and leaning forwards. I also have puffy swollen feet and ankles. My midwife has suggested I munch on as much parsley as possible to help with fluid loss. As I chomp down I feel like a cow, which is only reinforced by the fact that my boobs are now swollen full like udders! Ah, this new-mum phase—it's all glamour, isn't it? No!

I've decided today (Day 5) to walk my eldest boy to school with the new baby in the pram. It was only 10 minutes' easy stroll each way, but it felt like I climbed a mental mountain of just getting out of the house. I still feel quite wobbly, and the jelly belly is not helping. I'm doing my lower abdominals and pelvic floor exercises, but it takes a lot of concentration to switch them on. I've decided at my age (45) I'm going to be gentle but firm with my 'self-talk' about getting back into exercise again. I'm not as young as I used to be, that's a fact, but I'm definitely craving to be moving and back to my pre-pregnancy weight and shape. I'm committed to doing the small steps each week towards that goal. Oh, the broken sleep is just hell, isn't it? I'd forgotten how hard that is on your body.

Phase 1: 0–2 weeks (immediately post-birth)

Yes, everything feels incredibly flabby and mushy. You are wondering if you will ever lose your huge, wobbly belly, which has decreased a little post-birth but not as much as you would have thought, or liked! You may be a bit unsteady on your feet as you get used to not having that big bump out front. The pregnancy hormone relaxin which has helped loosen your body in preparation for the birth process is still present, but will gradually decrease over the next six months. However, for now you should exercise and move with care, as your ligaments, tendons and joints are relatively unsupported. In particular, repetitive bending, carrying, breastfeeding or bottle-feeding your baby will put increased strain on your back and neck. Add that to weakened ligaments and potentially poor posture, and you could be in the firing line for a sore back and neck. So, what to do?

Non-negotiable 1: pelvic floor exercises (PFs)

As discussed extensively in Chapter 3, these muscles are crucial for pelvic organ support and continence control (avoidance of urine leakage). If you have been exercising throughout your pregnancy, you will have been doing pelvic floor exercises and will be familiar with their function and importance.

After a vaginal delivery you can start doing PFs from day one; the sooner the better. The sling of pelvic floor muscles will have been extensively stretched, including the nerves that supply the area. You may be swollen, bruised and numb. If you have perineal damage, either through a planned cut (episiotomy) or through tearing, these exercises are beneficial as they bring improved blood flow to the wound and help both the vagina and perineum heal more quickly.

From day one, when you are either lying down or sitting on the toilet, think about the muscles and try to elicit even just a flicker of activity. Despite feeling like very little is happening initially, they will spring back into action relatively quickly, so just persist.

After a caesarean you can and should resume your PFs. Despite your baby's exit passage being via the sunroof, you have still had the weight of the baby pressing down on your pelvic floor during your final trimester, and this may have weakened the sling of muscles.

What to do

Squeeze and draw in and up around your anus (back passage), vagina and urethra (bladder outlet). Lift up inside and try to hold this contraction for as long as you can (3–5 seconds). Keep breathing! Now release and relax. Remember the PF mantra: **lift, squeeze, hold, relax.**

Frequency

Start with sets of 5–10 repetitions three times a day. You need to make these PFs a habit, so it is helpful to link doing them to something else you do repetitively, like breastfeeding, having a drink, or after each time you go to the toilet. Build up to doing 10 sets of 10 seconds every day. Add in some quick flick-type contractions, too.

> **TIP:** *I did PFs during the night feeds. The house was quiet, I'd get baby latched on for breastfeeding, make sure I was sitting supported and relaxed and then I'd do my sets of PFs. I had stitches from an episiotomy, but doing PFs wasn't painful; in fact, I think I healed quicker because of them.*

Check back to Chapter 3 for visualisations that will encourage you to perform sustained strong PF contractions. Remember the good form tips of not holding your breath, not pushing down, not pulling your abdominals in tightly and not tightening your buttocks and thighs.

Strong pelvic floor muscles mean you can exercise, cough, sneeze or laugh without the worry of leaking urine. Don't settle for anything less. If after your six-week postnatal check you can't tighten your muscles strongly, you are experiencing pain when you do so, or you are leaking urine, then make sure you ask for help from your doctor. It is likely that they will refer you to someone who specialises in helping women regain good pelvic floor activation. Get expert help now and avoid having continence problems in the future.

Non-negotiable 2: transverse abdominal exercises (TVAs)

For vaginal delivery you can start this exercise from day one or two. If you have had a caesarean section, wait one or two weeks for your wound to heal and then begin lower tummy tightening. (Your progress through the phases will be with an additional one to two weeks added on.)

Remember back to Chapter 4, where we discussed and introduced the various layers of abdominal muscles? Your priority in the first two weeks, and then extending through the phases, is to get the deepest layer (TVA) activated and working strongly again. This is the basis on which you will build a foundation of core strength that will give your body, and particularly your back, the necessary support it needs. I cannot over-emphasise how *important* it is to get this deep abdominal muscle working correctly to provide strong stability support now and for the rest of your life.

All of your abdominal muscles were stretched to accommodate your growing baby over the past nine months. The stretching is likely to have resulted in a gap between the edges of the muscle running down the centre of your abdominals—the fibrous line that stretches is called the linea alba, which is made of connective tissue, not muscle. The size of the gap (diastasis) varies depending on the size of the baby and the number of previous pregnancies, but it can be up to 5–10 finger-widths wide. The gap is not a hole, it is just stretched connective tissue, but it means that there is no longer strong muscular support on the front wall of your abdominals, thus it is an area of structural weakness that needs to be encouraged to shrink back to its original size.

Doing TVA exercises will help you achieve this. Working to get your TVA muscle back to its former glory is not just for looks, it's for functionality and to prevent potential back strain and pain. Your aim is to activate the TVA regularly (daily) to encourage the two sides of the abdominal muscles to pull together and to eliminate the gap, if not completely (ideal) then to no more than one finger-width. Activating and strengthening your TVA forms a solid platform which allows you to then progress on to other, more advanced, exercises and is the start of losing your post-pregnancy belly. The TVA is a major stabilising muscle, and you can think of it acting like an internal weight belt, whereas the more superficial abdominal muscles like the rectus abdominis is more responsible for definition.

Test for diastasis recti (abdominal separation)

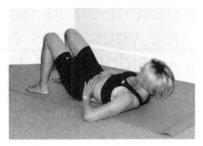

Lie on your back with your knees bent up and feet flat on floor. Place two fingers on your belly button and slide them down a few centimetres, then gently raise your head just off the floor. You will feel the stomach muscles tense, and what you need to feel for now is for the gap in between. Move your fingers back and forth, and side to side, to feel the extent of the gap. Gauge how big the gap is both in width and length. Between two and four finger-widths from the two edges of the abdominal muscle means you have a normal diastasis which still needs to shrink back. Four fingers or more means you have a fairly large gap, and you will need to adjust how you attempt abdominal exercises initially to encourage this gap to narrow. Using your arms crossed across your body to encourage the two edges of the muscle together can provide additional support.

Make a mental note of the size of the gap at this point so you can monitor how it shrinks back together with your practice of regular TVA exercises over the next 12 weeks. Don't sit up when you finish the test, especially if you have just identified a decent-sized gap. Instead, roll to the side and use your arms to push yourself up into a sitting position, and remember to do this until you have shrunk the stretched gap.

What to do

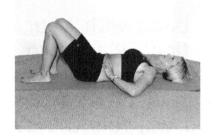

Fig.8.1

Lying on your back, with your knees bent up and your feet flat on the ground, think about drawing your tummy muscles in and down towards the floor. Suck your belly button towards your spine. Keep breathing evenly. As with your initial efforts with your pelvic floor muscles, it may feel as if nothing is happening, but even if the activation is small, just keep persisting. The nerves will send the necessary messages to the muscle and it will increasingly respond over the next few days, providing you keep doing the exercise regularly. Remember: use it or lose it.

If you need further reinforcement that you are doing the right sort of contraction, then feel the muscle activate by pressing your fingers on the inside of your hip bones. If you then cough you will feel the muscle fibres of TVA bounce up against your fingers. It is important to remember to *brace* this muscle—pull it in and down. Remember the 'zip it up' analogy from Chapter 4? Think now of zipping up your pelvic floor and zipping in your abdominals from either side, so that you now have firm, braced support across your lower abdomen.

You can also turn on your TVA in four-point kneeling. Put one hand on your belly and suck your bellybutton upwards towards your spine.

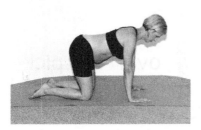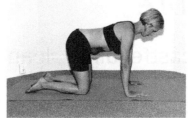

Fig.8.2

Frequency

During Phase 1 do your TVAs two to three times a day. While you may initially find it easier to do them in a lying position, you can also try them while standing or sitting. Basically, wherever you are and whenever you remember, do a set. At the very least, when you get into bed at night do some long, sustained holds, beginning with 10–30 seconds at a time. So a minimum would be five lots of 30 seconds, two to three times a day.

TIP: *In your sleep-deprived state you may need to remind yourself to do these important two exercises. Write 'PF and TVA' as a visual reminder and stick a note on the fridge. Ask your partner to remind you to do them. Doing these two non-negotiables frequently in the first two weeks is the key to getting back on track.*

The final two things to consider and include in Phase 1 are posture and pram walks.

Posture

Breastfeeding, leaning over to pick up or put down baby, and carrying your little bundle all add up to a lot of forward flexion in these first few weeks. Weakened ligaments, tight, sore muscles from hours sitting breastfeeding, and general tiredness mean your posture can tend to be poor. Poor posture can cause back and neck aches.

Sit in a supported upright position and drop your shoulders down and back when breastfeeding or bottle-feeding your baby. Think of sliding your shoulder blades back together. You will spend a lot of your day and night sitting while feeding your baby, so it is worth getting your posture right.

Regularly do a cat-style stretch. On the floor, kneeling with your arms extended out in front of you, your butt lifted high, pull back from your fingertips and press your chest down. Rest your forehead on the floor and feel the stretch through your shoulders, chest and back.

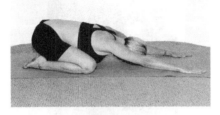

Fig.8.3

A tendency in these first few months is to unconsciously elevate one or both of your shoulders while you are lifting, carrying and holding your baby. You'll probably be doing the normal thing a mum does: baby held with one arm as you use your other hand to do incredible one-handed manoeuvres. Over time that can lead to sustained muscle tension and pain in your upper back and neck. There is no point saying don't do it, as this is just how mums need to operate, so the best advice is to be aware that when you lift and hold baby like this you should keep your shoulders down and your head and neck in a neutral position. Check every now and again, and do a quick shoulder drop. Another good mobilisation action is to gently do rotational spine twists either when standing or sitting, or sitting on a Swiss ball.

Pram walks

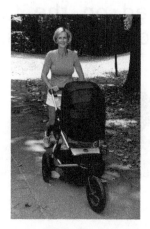

Fig.8.4

Getting out and walking with your baby in a pram around your local neighbourhood is something that is not only good for your circulation but good for your mental health, too. It can feel like an endless cycle of sleep (or not!), feeding, nappy changes, etc., so getting a breath of fresh air and a change of scenery can do you the world of good.

Your walk doesn't have to be long in duration, and flat terrain is best in these first few weeks. Something is better than nothing. You will be able to build on both duration and intensity in the coming weeks.

TIP: *I was lent a bassinet attachment for my mountain buggy which was great as I could go for a walk with baby sleeping comfortably in a horizontal position. A good pram for exercise-walking has soft inflatable tyres with a bassinet attachment. Anything that helps you get out the door and exercise in the fresh air is a decent investment in your health and wellbeing.*

Dear Diary—Week 2

It's working! After a week of daily TVAs, I'm noticing a difference. Practice makes ... well not perfect, but it's certainly a start in the right direction.

I am now living through a foggy haze of sleep deprivation. This week I'm going for longer walks, but still at a very relaxed pace. My legs feel stronger. I really get relief for my tight upper back if I do a cat stretch on the floor. I can't live without my support knickers at the moment—they hold in my tummy and all that excess skin! Will it ever shrink?

Tips and insights for Phase 1

✳ Consider using a pillow under your knee when lying on your side in bed. You may have slept like this in the latter stages of pregnancy, too, but it is worth continuing on for a few weeks at least, as it will ensure your pelvis and spine are in a comfortable neutral position.

✳ If you can organise it (and get babysitting cover), getting a massage is a wonderful treat in these first few weeks. It is especially relieving for niggles, twinges and aches you can experience as your body adjusts.

✳ If you endured a particularly arduous birthing process, you may wish to consider a visit to an osteopath to check alignment of your pelvis. Getting this checked early on can help you avoid ongoing pelvis or back problems.

✳ If you are breastfeeding, you are likely to have heavier, fuller breasts. Make sure for walking and any upcoming exercising you have a properly sized, fully supportive bra. To provide enough support you may need to wear an exercise bra underneath, then a firm-fitting lycra bra over the top.

✳ If your bleeding (lochia) becomes heavier, this may be sign you are overdoing things, so back off and check with your LMC.

✳ You may wish to wear a belly band (wide elasticised belt) or some sort of firm wrap of material around your abdominal region for the first two to six weeks. Adding some external support will act as a reminder to tighten and brace your lower abdominal region, and the feeling of support you get will eventually be replaced by your own reactivated TVA.

* Be very careful when lifting any sort of load during your first six weeks of recovery. The normal strength that would come from your abdominals and back is diminished due to your weakened stretched tummy region, and until you have strengthened your TVA to provide bracing support you must take particular care. One action that you are likely to be doing frequently is lifting the baby capsule in and out of the car. This involves lifting, twisting and bending forwards; the combination of which can spell high risk of injury. Ideally get someone else to do this sort of lifting if at all possible; if it's not, then before you begin, consciously brace and switch on your lower abdominals, holding the capsule close and making the movement as smooth and controlled as possible. Breaking the task down into several stages and stabilising as you go means you are less likely to risk a back strain.

* By 12 weeks your baby may weigh close to 6 kilograms, add in the capsule weight and you have got a hefty load to be moving around. Be careful early on and save yourself the pain of a strain.

Remember: Be kind to yourself. Get as much sleep as you can. Realise that life will get easier as your baby gets into a routine. Know that your body *will* recover and that you are on the right track. Hang in there, new mum—you are doing great!

✓ Do daily PFs and TVAs.

✓ Remember good posture.

✓ Get out for a pram walk whenever you can—no pace, just grace!

Phase 2: 2–6 weeks (until your postnatal check)

By now you will hopefully have begun regular PFs and TVAs. If for whatever reason you haven't been able to, then you really need to spend a week practising regular activation before you progress on. They are simply the non-negotiables, and if you don't start them now then you will have to go back to these basic exercises at some stage in the future. This next month or so with your baby is still very tiring and time-consuming, so if you are finding it impossible to get any time to exercise then consider two things:

1. You can do the non-negotiables (PFs and TVAs) when you are actually doing other things. They are perfect exercises for multitasking and we all know how brilliant females are at doing that! Try them when

feeding baby, when standing at the kitchen sink, etc.

2. You will need to make a conscious decision to make exercise (even the bare minimum) something of a priority in this new-baby busy-mum existence. There is plenty of research that confirms that slotting in some exercise time can be super-beneficial in these weeks when you are recovering. You probably don't need me to remind you that *yes, you are still recovering.* The right sort of exercise can: improve your strength and stamina, which makes looking after your new baby a little easier; give you more energy, not less, providing you don't overdo it; and bring about a positive frame of mind.

Just make sure you are filling up your 'rest tank' before you attempt exertion. By sleeping when the baby sleeps, or at least getting horizontal, you are stocking up your rest tank and fuelling your ability to do some meaningful exercise. Your order of priority for the first six weeks is to boost your rest tank first, with exercise to follow.

Exercises

Pelvic floor exercises

Continue on with the pelvic floor exercises, but increase the squeeze intensity. Lift up, squeeze and hold for 10 seconds, then slowly release. Do 10 repetitions, then 10 quick flick contractions, squeeze and release.

TVA progression—TVA plus leg slides

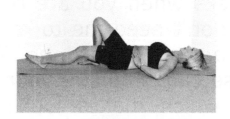

Fig.8.5

Add a leg slide to the static (or holding) TVA contraction. Do a couple of 30-second static holds to begin with, then with your lower abdominals pulled in and zipped up, slowly slide one leg flat to the floor. This move requires a more intense contraction of your lower abdominals. Bend your leg back up to the starting position. Continue alternate leg sliding, lowering down and up, 2 seconds down, 2 seconds up, and complete 10 with each leg. Your lower back should be held in a neutral position throughout, not arched or pressed flat to the floor. There should be just enough hollow space to slide one hand in under your lower back. Alternate (superset) this with a set of bridging lifts (see Fig.8.7).

Beginner butt activation

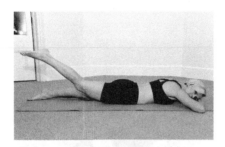

Fig.8.6

Lying on your stomach (use a pillow under your ribcage for comfort if you have full or tender breasts), squeeze both buttocks together first before you move anything, then with a straight leg lift one heel up as far as you can, squeezing your butt continuously. Don't twist your hips to get higher—it's meant to be a small-range movement. Then lower your leg while still contracting the muscle—once you can feel your thigh back on the floor, you can let go and relax the muscle. Do 10 on each leg, doing three sets, slowly and with control.

This exercise is important for re-educating the correct muscle-firing pattern for the butt region which may have altered during pregnancy. Rest your fingers on your butt cheeks to check that the muscle is squeezed tight. Once you are able to perform this exercise with ease, then progress to bridging (overleaf). From now on start to consciously think of switching on your buttock muscles

432

when walking up stairs, walking up any inclines, pushing the pram, etc.

Bridging

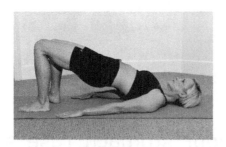

Fig.8.7

This exercise is called 'bridging' because you are making a bridge shape with your body. While on your back, with your knees bent in, squeeze your butt muscles tightly and then lift your butt up as high as you can, keeping your hips level. It is important at this stage to perform the exercise in this order: squeeze and contract the butt muscles first, and then lift up. The reason for pre-contracting the muscle is that the normal pattern of butt muscle activation is likely to have been altered (weakened) due to your pregnancy, particularly in the third trimester when you were probably walking with a waddle due to your expanded shape. If you do this exercise as prescribed, you will be re-educating your butt muscles to switch on and activate in the proper sequence when required. Back pain and injury post-pregnancy can often be traced back to weak, deactivated butt muscles, thus a bit of focus and persistence now in getting this sequence right will pay dividends as you progress with more active pursuits. So squeeze, then lift and hold for 10 seconds, and lower. Repeat 10 times. Complete three sets of each exercise.

Half-side-planks

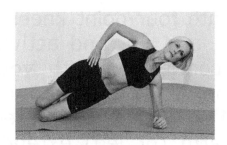

Fig.8.8

Roll onto your side, with knees bent in, then press up on your elbow into a half-side-plank position, and lift your hips up off the floor. Hold for 5–10 seconds initially, building up to five 30-second lift holds. Start with the free hand resting lightly in front of you on the floor for balance, but move that onto your upper thigh as you improve your balance in this position. Roll to the other side and complete the exercises.

Three-point kneeling holds

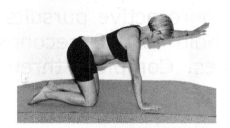

Fig.8.9

Turn over into four-point kneeling, draw your belly button in and up, and activate your TVA. Maintain the contraction with your spine in a neutral position as you extend each limb out (1 x L arm, 1 x R arm, 1 x R leg, 1 x L leg) holding each arm (or leg) extended for a few seconds, and then returning it to the original four-point kneeling position. Go around the four limbs three times. (Again, remember to squeeze and activate the butt muscle *before* extending the leg.) Draw back into a cat stretch to finish, and hold for 30–60 seconds.

Seated rows with exercise band

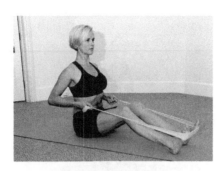

Fig.8.10

Using some form of stretch resistance (band or cable), sit with your knees slightly bent, and loop the band around both feet. Drop your shoulders down and, using an underhand grip, draw your elbows back towards your ribs. As you draw the ends of the band towards your body, squeeze between your shoulder blades. Pause and release slowly. Complete 15 repetitions in a slow rhythm. Squeeze in for 2 seconds, hold for 2 seconds, release for 2 seconds.

Single standing knee-bends

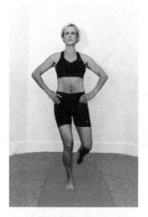

Fig.8.11

Standing on one leg (L), keep your hips bones even and level throughout (visualise having headlights on your hip bones and keep the beams pointing forwards). Rest your hands on your hips, thumbs on your pelvis bones and fingers pressing in, to check you are activating your TVA throughout. Bend the L knee directly forward over your toe, with your upper body staying vertical, and importantly your pelvis staying level as you complete the movement. Perform 10 slow and controlled repetitions, then repeat on the R leg. Initially, you may find it helpful to watch in full-length mirror so you can ensure neither hip is tilting or dropping. It may seem a very simple movement, but the key is in turning on the abdominals and the butt muscles to keep your pelvis stable while balancing on one leg. It involves the crucial core muscles that, when strengthened, will allow you to resume more strenuous exercising safely and without risk of lower back strain or injury.

Pram walk extension (i)

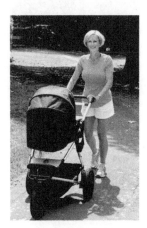

Fig.8.12

Now you can start increasing the duration of your walks to 30–60 minutes, including gentle undulating terrain. See if you can manage three or more walks a week.

TVA on the move
When out walking, choose a nominal distance—one or three lampposts, for example—and activate your TVA as you are walking that distance. Put your hands on your hips, press inside your hip bone to feel your TVA brace and support. Suck your belly button towards your spine, hold for the lamppost distance. Build to three or more, keep your breathing rhythmical, and your shoulders down

and relaxed. Doing this, you are activating the TVA in a functional way.

Body weight squats, static lunges and standing wall presses

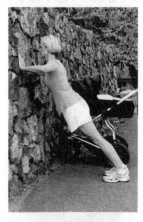

Fig.8.13

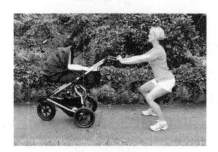

Fig.8.14

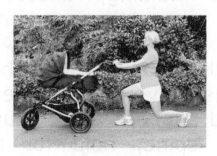

Fig.8.15

While you are on your walk I want you to add in a few other exercises as you go. Have three pauses on your walk to complete these three exercises in a circuit.

√ 15 x squats (squeeze the butt first, then rise up).

√ 10 x lunges on each leg (squeeze the butt first, then rise up).

√ 10 wall presses—the further back your feet, the harder it will be. Maintain a straight plank body position. Focus on using your chest muscle to push back.

Dear Diary—Week 3

I've had some upper back pain and some neck pain. I know it's definitely due to all the breastfeeding and lifting of baby, but it has eased quite a bit with the stretches and mobilising I have done. My tummy is shrinking and I'm feeling stronger. Today I did my TVAs while out in the car, and I also did some when settling baby at night, kneeling beside the bassinet. I have to consciously remind myself to activate my TVA every time I lift baby out of the bassinet. He's getting heavier each week, too; stacking on the kilos, which is a good thing. I am noticing that breastfeeding really saps your energy, so I need to make sure I eat well. YAY for heat-and-eat meals. I'm glad I made the effort in those last few weekends before baby arrived to cook up a storm and stock the freezer with casseroles and lasagnes. The last thing I feel like doing at 6pm is cooking a meal from scratch. I need to make sure I don't overdo the walking; I think I might have pushed it a bit today. I must take it easy for the next few days.

When things are going well, in that I've managed to breastfeed, burp and get baby settled and off to sleep again, I feel slightly euphoric as if I've achieved something major. I'm trying to read his tired signs. I find I'm spending an extraordinary amount of time each day trying to get his burps up!

Tips and insights for Phase 2

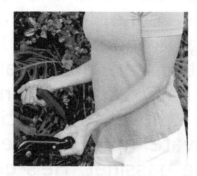

Fig.8.16

✳ Pushing the pram up an incline can be really hard work. Make sure your effort is generated primarily from your core abdominal region by using an underhand grip or ensuring your elbows are back drawn in beside your ribs. These two adjustments make you use your core to generate the pushing motion. Be standing as upright as possible as you walk, not leaning forward and rounding your back.

✳ Remember to consciously reactivate your butt muscles in these early weeks. By practising squeezing the butt first before doing exercises like squats, lunges and walking up stairs, you will be re-establishing and reinforcing the correct muscle firing pattern. After a few weeks it becomes automatic, and you won't have to think about it; then you'll know that your gluts will activate as required to provide necessary support. An underperforming butt region can cause excess strain on your back and hamstrings and potentially lead to injury.

✳ If you find it difficult to get time to do the exercises in one block, split them so that you do some in the morning and some at night. The simple fact is that fitting exercise in during this time as a new mum takes determination and a good dose of compromise. Just do what you can when you can, and praise yourself for doing it. There will be days when it simply is not possible. Remember tomorrow is another day and another chance to slot in some exercise. You may find you develop tightness on one side of your body (the side flexor muscles around your ribs) due to repeatedly holding your baby on one side. As well as stretching your shoulders and chest area, add in some side stretches when standing; lying sideways supported over a Swiss ball can also alleviate tightness.

Programme plan

√ Home exercises numbers 1–6 daily, or at least every second day.

√ Pram walk with exercises three times a week.

√ Stretches: Focus on tight upper-body muscles with a particular emphasis on opening out your chest, shoulder circles backwards, and stretching your neck by dropping your ear down towards your shoulder either side.

Phase 3: 6–12 weeks (onwards and upwards)

Dear Diary—Week 6

I've hit the wall. It's taken until now for the post-birth high to wear off and the cumulative tiredness to stack up. I'm knackered. It's meant to be a particularly 'sunny period' with baby according to the developmental books, but he's cranky and hard to settle. I can't find time for a nap for me during the day, so exercise is becoming hard to achieve. The weekends are easier when I can offload baby minding onto my hubby. When I do some exercise I feel great—my body is craving it. On Saturday I did a cycle on the stationary bike at home, and on Sunday I did toning exercises and stretches. Bliss. It made a nice change from walking. Variety is the key for me, and just getting something in rather than nothing. I thought in the first few weeks that I'd never feel like the old me again, but slowly and surely my muscle strength is coming back—even amidst the exhaustion. This motherhood role is SO busy, and it's pretty much a monotonous cycle at present of: feed baby; burp baby; change baby; settle baby to sleep; do a load of washing or grab a nap or get some domestic chores done. Looking after a new baby is a responsible full-time job with loads of unpredictable demands. Multi-tasking is the only way I can fit everything in. I'm now doing the walk-to-school drop-off, and then continuing on for a longer pram walk while baby sleeps, with exercises out and about as I go. I felt a little self-conscious initially about doing the wall press-ups on someone else's wall, but that lasted a nanosecond. Passengers in the cars driving by must have wondered what I was doing—ha ha!

Exercises

Pelvic floor exercises

This goes without saying by now, right? Good! Get into the habit of doing a PF pull-up every time you activate your TVA.

TVA progression—TVA plus toe touches

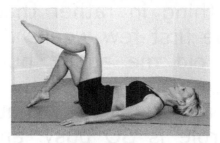

Fig.8.17

The next progression to further strengthen your TVA is performed lying on your back, with both knees pulled in and feet off the floor. Maintain a static TVA contraction and slowly lower alternate toes to lightly touch the floor, then lift up again, and repeat 15 times with each leg.

Step-ups

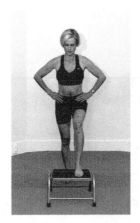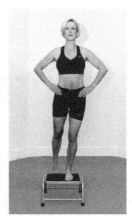

Fig.8.18

Using either the stairs, your front doorstep or a box that is stable to stand on, do a set of step-ups on each leg. Your left leg stays on the step as you rise up and down, and then do the same with the right. The key to this exercise is to activate your butt first, before your leg muscles, so before you step up, squeeze your butt. Make sure that as you step up you keep your bent knee tracking straight forwards, over your toe (not rolling in). Put your hands on your butt cheeks as if you were putting them in your back pockets, to check that the muscle is activating and staying contracted throughout the movement.

Bridging with single leg extension

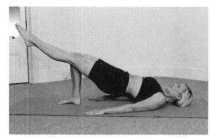

Fig.8.19

Squeeze your butt, lift and perform a bridge, then slowly extend one leg out whilst maintaining your lifted level pelvis position. You will need to switch on your core muscles strongly (abdominals and gluteals) to perform this slowly and smoothly while keeping your hip bones even. Extend your lower leg out, hold for 3 seconds, and return to original position. Continue with alternate single leg extensions, and repeat 15 times on each side.

Side-lying planks progression plus side leg-lifts

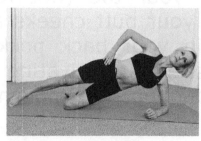

Fig.8.20

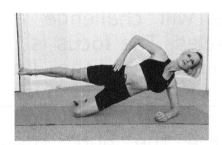

Fig.8.21

Perform a side-lying plank as in Phase 2, lifting your hips up (Fig.8.20. While in this position, lift and lower your hip to the floor, in pulses. Extend your upper leg (Fig.8.21); hold the half-plank position while doing a set of upper leg-lifts for outer-thigh strengthening. This exercise targets two sets of muscles: the obliques are activated by the side plank position, and the leg abductors are activated on the upper side. Don't lift the upper leg too high: just elevate it in line with your body, no higher than your shoulder, and toe pointing down. Complete 15–20 repetitions each side.

Alternate two-point kneeling holds

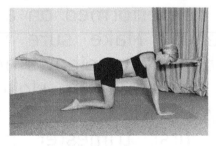

Fig.8.22

Again, this will challenge and strengthen your core muscles. The focus is to maintain the hips and shoulders in the kneeling neutral position—don't sway or move to the side. Activate TVA first by drawing in your belly button. Squeeze the butt, then extend the opposite arm and leg, hold for 3 seconds, then pull them in to under your body, not touching the floor, and begin to extend again. Complete 10 repetitions on the one side, and then return to four-point kneeling. Complete the same exercise with the other arm and leg: extend, draw in, extend, etc.

Tricep dips

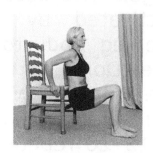

Fig.8.23

These can be performed on a step, a chair or a park bench. Make sure your chest is vertical, then bend your elbows and lower your body, keeping your butt as close to the step or chair as you can. (This is the same as exercise 5 in first trimester home workout session.) You can advance the exercise by extending one leg out. Do a set of 10–15 repetitions.

These first seven exercises can be performed in a circuit. Aim for 2 sets of each.

Single knee-bends plus knee-repeater

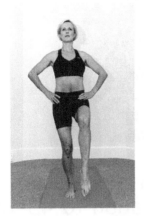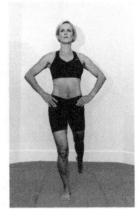

Fig.8.24

Perform the knee-bending exercise as instructed in the Phase 2 programme, but increase to 20 repetitions. Then, staying balanced on the same leg, extend your other leg backwards for a set of 20 knee-repeaters. Keep your pelvis still and level by drawing in your TVA to provide strong, braced core support

Pram walk extension (ii)

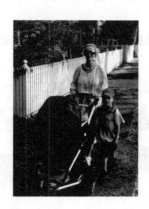

Add some hills and undulating terrain to your walks. Increase duration to 45–60 minutes, or longer if you feel up to it. Increase to a brisk-paced walk. Continue with doing three pauses for squats, walking lunges and wall press-outs.

Squat holds, alternate walking lunges and wall press-outs

√ **Squat holds** Legs slightly wider than hip-distance apart, toes turned out. Squat down and hold for 3 seconds, then squeeze the butt and rise. 20 repetitions, 3 sets.

√ **Alternate walking lunges** Press your fingers into your butt muscles to check that they are contracting throughout. 15 each leg (30 total per set), 3 sets.

√ **Wall press-outs** Angle your body more by having your feet further away. Activate your TVA to maintain a straight plank position with your body as you perform the exercise. 20 repetitions, 3 sets.

Dear Diary—Week 9

Oh, bless the almighty burp! I never thought I'd be so fixated on the production of a burp, or rather a cluster of burps. Burp production seems to determine the tone of my day in this first 12 weeks. A series of plentiful burps post a feed means I get a calm baby who's easy to settle, and therefore I can actually get a few things done in the brief sleep window. If there are no burps then I get an unsettled, grimacing baby, and I can kiss goodbye to any 'me' time. Thus long live the humble BURP!

Tips and insights for Phase 3

* It is likely that you will still feel twinges and aches in odd parts of your body as the pregnancy hormones that have allowed laxity in the ligaments that support your joints gradually dissipate. Try to build towards three to five exercise sessions a week, whether at home or out and about. Aim to complete the exercises, but it's okay if you don't always get there. Something is better than nothing. Split the session up if that is easier: 15 minutes in the morning, 15 minutes at night, and PFs and TVAs lying in front of television.

* If you haven't already done so, consider meeting up with another mum who's at a similar stage with her baby, and do pram walks together. This may or may not work depending on each baby's feeding routine, but it can be motivating to have an exercise buddy. You can always reward yourselves with a chat and coffee at a café as the conclusion of your walking workout. Keep listening to your body, and balance your exercise and rest needs. This is not a time to push yourself hard, as you are still recovering from giving birth.

* If you want to resume classes at a gym, find out if there are any postnatal options, or choose classes that are not high-impact, and modify the movements accordingly. For example, cycle classes can be a good start as you can set you own level of intensity. Resistance or weight workouts should be at about 50% of pre-pregnancy level. Until your TVA is strong and you have little or no abdominal gap (diastasis), refrain from doing any planks, sit-ups, etc. Find out what crèche facilities your local gym may offer.

* Aqua aerobics or swimming are good options, providing you have had seven days without any bleeding or discharge from your vagina and any wounds are fully healed. Pilates and yoga are also great, as they focus on the core and are low-impact. Tell the class teacher how many weeks postpartum you are.

  * Stationary cycle, treadmill or the stepper are also excellent options for getting some beneficial cardiovascular exercise. Getting a sweat up can feel really good and it won't affect your breast milk's quality or quantity. Ease back into it, and work at about 50–75% intensity. The perceived exertion level should be 'somewhat hard', not hard. Buying or renting a piece of cardio exercise equipment can make it easier to fit in workouts at home around your new baby or other children.

  * Resuming running at this phase still poses some jarring risks for your back, especially if your TVA and butt strength is not yet able to support strong, single-leg pelvic stability. Heavy breasts and loose joints can make this form of impact exercise uncomfortable. It is preferable to wait until at least 12 weeks before hitting the pavements again, and when you do: build up slowly. To test whether your TVA activation is automatically providing sufficient pelvic stability for running, in front of a mirror perform a set of one-legged knee-bends, with your hands identifying the crest of your pelvis bones either side. If (without you consciously trying) your pelvis stays level throughout the bending

motion, then it's likely you are strong enough to begin to ease back into running. If, however, there is any tilting (however small), you need to continue to strengthen your TVAs with both bracing and exercises as outlined in this chapter. The running motion means you are shifting your entire body weight side to side as you heel strike, with increased flexion and rotational forces on your spine. If you are not fully strong and supported through your pelvis, then your back will take the strain and you may end up with muscle spasm or injury. Be patient and get strong before adding impact.

* You may find some of your pre-pregnancy clothing fits you now, so you can take a break from those well-worn stretchy track pants and loose tops. Now might even be a good time to buy something new as a reward for all the hard work you have been putting in with baby, family and your progressive return to fitness.

Dear Diary—Week 10

I've now managed to get to the gym once or twice a week, thanks to my hubby babysitting and also the gym's crèche. I've started with RPM (cycle class) and some of my own weight training, but everything is quite modified. I was a bit sore for a few days after the first couple of sessions, but it's a good sort of muscle soreness. I'm doing my specific TVA strengthening before or after class. My body is clearly still adapting to the change from pregnancy to new mum.

I'm gradually increasing the cardio intensity, but I'm not pushing hard as I'm still breastfeeding and I'm very aware of the energy that's taking, plus I haven't caught up on my sleep deprivation yet from the first nine weeks. Each week it's getting better and better. I'm glad I'm through that hard brand-new baby stage, as he's now in a routine most of the time and I'm getting regular exercise. It's onwards and upwards from here.

Phase 4: 12+ weeks (resuming regular exercise)

Be mindful that the hormones that caused necessary joint laxity during pregnancy and birth can stay present in lessening amounts in your system for up to six months, so some caution and care are still necessary from 12 weeks postpartum. However, in general you will feel like and be able to resume more vigorous exercise. Now that you are regularly doing PFs contractions (continue for life) and your TVA is providing strong, bracing support for your back and pelvis, you can gradually introduce the sort of exercising you preferred pre-pregnancy. You can now do sit-ups or curl-ups as part of your abdominal exercises.

For continuing weight loss and fitness goals, make sure each week you have three or four targeted cardiovascular workouts of 30–60 minutes' duration, and gradually increase your intensity. Check out the low impact class options at your local gym or community centre. BODYVIVE™ (a Les Mills group fitness programme) is an all-round low-impact workout which is ideal for postnatal mums. General muscle strengthening, using weights or body weight as resistance, is also important as part of a balanced overall programme. Gaining lean muscle tissue means you become more of a fat-burning machine.

As your baby grows, they naturally get heavier. The repeated carrying and lifting will put stress on your back, so it is important to continue with regular TVA maintenance exercises, and definitely switch them on prior to doing any other more advanced abdominal strengthening work. Also include exercises like lateral pull-downs and seated rows to ensure you are strengthening your back so that it is able to withstand the increasing strain, and consciously switch on your butt muscles when doing exercises like squats, lunges and step-ups to maintain power and control in your lower body.

Some mums report still feeling muscle and joint twinges and niggles many months postnatal, not only during the first 12 weeks. This is quite normal and just part of the body easing itself back after pregnancy. Keep listening to your body and adjusting and modifying your exercise programme as necessary to accommodate this.

Priorities and positives

It will always be a juggle between motherhood and time for exercising, especially for mums who are over 35. Once you have a child (or two, or three) that's always the case, but gym crèche facilities and choosing exercise activities that the family can participate in at the weekend (beach walks or tramping, for example) are just two suggestions from a range of planning options you will need to employ in order to get that valuable time to keep yourself healthy. A fit, healthy and therefore happy mum has more energy to devote to her family and is better able to keep a robust resilience in the face of never-ending calls on your time from little ones.

Research offers some other incentives to get back into action. Studies have shown that moderate exercise can boost your mood.

Furthermore, research has looked at whether exercising postpartum can alleviate postnatal depression (PND). Although not definitive, there have been signs of decreased incidence of PND, but only if exercise is performed at a moderate intensity level—not hard.

Butt, butt and ... more butt

You may think that I have written a lot about firing up your butt muscles as part of your postnatal recovery and resumption of exercise. There is a definite reason for this, based on personal experience. I got a painful injury at 14 weeks postnatally because my gluteals weren't firing equally or correctly. I sought assessment and, through having to rehabilitate myself, I gained a thorough appreciation of the importance for new mums to retrain and strengthen this particular area.

Most of us sit more in our daily lives, so we generally use our buttock muscles less. Pregnancy alters your shape and posture, so again the buttock muscles are switched off most of the time. Yet the buttock muscles play a very important role in supporting the body's core region, as well as initiating and supporting lower-body movement. Most postnatal mums will have weak buttock muscles, despite doing squats and exercising appropriately during pregnancy. Now is the time for you to switch them on again, and the best way to do that is through a structured, progressive strengthening programme where you are retraining your brain to stimulate the correct movement pattern. You need to be patient and persevere. Retraining a muscle firing pattern to become a habit takes a matter of weeks (about three to six weeks) with constant awareness and repetitive effort. It is well worth putting in the effort now, as once you have re-established the correct muscle firing pattern it will become automatic. If you miss the opportunity to focus on this now, then you run the risk of getting injuries as you progress to more regular exercising, because the muscles won't be kicking in as they should. If you find it difficult to activate the buttock muscles or are unsure how to get them firing in the exercises in this chapter, then I highly recommend you go and see a physiotherapist to help you get started correctly. The preference would be to pick a therapist who specialises in musculoskeletal rehabilitation.

Nutrition and weight loss

The first 12 weeks postpartum is not the time to diet, nor is it a time to indulge with every sweet, sticky treat you can lay your hands on. If you resume eating a sensible diet within the principles of balance, variety and moderation, combined with the exercises as prescribed in this chapter, then you will be right on track to losing your pregnancy weight. Of course, if you have had another child in the past few years and didn't manage to lose that pregnancy weight, then keep your expectations realistic. One step at a time. Aim for slow, gradual weight loss, as the weight is more likely to stay off and it is safer for you and your baby. In order to achieve any weight loss from this pregnancy, or those before, adopt a sensible, healthy eating plan.

If you are breastfeeding, you must maintain enough energy intake to provide your baby with the nourishment they need through breast milk, plus your own body's calorific requirements.

If your baby is continuing to feed well and is putting on weight at a normal rate, you are including some regular moderate exercise in your weekly routine and being sensible about eating the right sort of foods in the right sort of amounts, then you have all the ingredients for achieving your weight loss goal.

How much can you lose? Up to half a kilogram a week is recommended for sensible, long-term weight loss.

> *If you follow a sensible diet, plus you are breastfeeding and exercising regularly, the research shows you'll experience weight loss three times faster than those mums who don't monitor their food intake.*

Healthy eating guidelines for breastfeeding, exercising mums

Mums who are exercising but not breastfeeding should also follow these healthy eating guidelines but will generally require fewer calories, so cut back on the portions/servings but maintain the variety.

Eat a variety from each of the four main food groups every day:

1. **Vegetables and fruit** provide carbohydrates (sugar and starch), fibre, vitamins and minerals, and are low in fat. Aim for plenty of colour in your daily repertoire of this food group. Go easy on fruit juice and dried fruits, which have a high sugar content. As a guide, have at least six servings a day of vegetables and fruit, broken down into at least four servings of vegetables and two servings of fruit.

2. **Breads and cereals** provide carbohydrates (sugar and starch), fibre, and nutrients such as B vitamins and minerals. Examples of healthy choices are brown rice, wholemeal pasta, low-sugar breakfast cereals, and other wholegrain products. Opt for wholegrain varieties because they provide extra nutrients and fibre which is good for bowel function. As a guide, have

approximately seven servings of this food group a day.

3. **Milk and milk products** (like yogurt and cheese) are a valuable source of protein vitamins and minerals, especially calcium and iodine, while breastfeeding. Preferably go for the reduced-fat or low-fat options. If you are drinking soy milk, choose one that is calcium-fortified. Have at least three servings a day of this food group.

4. **Lean meat, chicken, seafood, eggs, legumes, nuts and seeds** provide protein, iron, zinc and other nutrients. Choose at least two servings from this food group each day.

As a guide, a serving portion is approximately the size of your clenched fist.

As well as the four food groups above, there are some other important food factors to consider during this time.

Fluid

Aim for at least 10 cups of fluid each day. Breastfeeding will increase your fluid needs, as will hot weather and exercising. Make it a habit to drink a glass of water every time you feed your baby.

Coffee and tea

Moderate your intake, as you did during pregnancy, since caffeine is transferred to breast milk and could potentially make your baby unsettled. A suitable maximum level of consumption is no more than six cups of tea, or one double espresso coffee per day. Refer back to Chapter 2 for more detail on the caffeine levels found in common beverages.

Cut down, not out

Follow sensible healthy eating principles of cutting down on saturated fat, salt and sugar. It's fine to have treat foods and takeaways *occasionally,* just not frequently.

Supplements

You may choose to take a vitamin and mineral supplement while breast-feeding, as your nutritional requirements during this time are elevated. In particular, iodine is an essential nutrient required in small amounts to support normal growth and development including normal brain development. It is important that babies receive enough iodine. Foods that are sources of iodine include well-cooked seafood, milk, eggs, some cereals and commercially made bread. However, even with a well-balanced diet, it is difficult to get enough iodine from food alone. It is recommended that you take an iodine-specific supplement to give you approximately 270 micrograms a day during the time that you are breastfeeding. It may be included in a general pregnancy and breastfeeding multivitamin. If you have any concerns about your dietary intake, check with your doctor or dietician. As discussed in Chapter 2, vegetarian mums need to be very careful about getting the right balance of nutrients, especially when breastfeeding. Discuss how to ensure you are doing this with your doctor, and seek advice from specialist sources, such as the Vegetarian Society. (Similarly, if you are planning on raising your child on a vegetarian diet, you need to be vigilant that their nutritional requirements are met at *all* stages of development.)

Snack attack

It's important in the first three months of breastfeeding not to go too long without eating, ideally no longer than three to four hours, so have a stash of nutritious snacks on hand. Some snack ideas: roasted unsalted almonds, fruit, cheese and crackers, rice cakes, crumpets, pita bread, muffins, yogurt, vegetable sticks with cottage cheese or peanut butter, simple sandwiches, smoothies and creamed rice.

Breastfeeding

Effect of exercise

Research has shown that exercise does not affect the quality or quantity of breast milk produced; however, the only exception to this is for those women exercising at the absolute upper end of the intensity scale, doing anaerobic exercise where lactic acid is a metabolic by-product. In such cases the breast milk produced immediately after such an intense exercise session was described as 'somewhat changed in taste'. If you have exercised particularly hard for some reason, wait about an hour before breastfeeding, to minimise any potential change to your breast milk.

Most women who continue to exercise are back to their pre-conception weight within a year of giving birth. Some will lose their pregnancy weight more quickly than others. Breastfeeding can help some women with initial weight loss, with others it may be after you finish nursing your baby that you find it easier to lose those extra few kilos.

Alcohol

You have been off the alcohol for the past nine months, and now you face another stretch of abstinence while breastfeeding, as alcohol passes very quickly into breast milk and can negatively affect your baby, especially in the first few months. However, if you do choose to have an occasional glass or two, then you can minimise the risk of exposing your baby to it by waiting until the alcohol level in your breast milk has dropped. As an approximate guideline, after drinking alcohol wait from two to three

466

hours before resuming breastfeeding. If your baby needs to be fed during this time, you can offer previously expressed breast milk that is free from alcohol. You may wish to build up a supply in the freezer ahead of time. If you are expressing within two to three hours of drinking alcohol, you should discard the breast milk; pump and dump!

In closing...

Good luck with your ongoing health and wellbeing. You have traversed and negotiated the tough and physically challenging but incredibly rewarding journey of motherhood. Keeping fit and healthy is not rocket science, but it does involve a daily discipline of keeping exercise and good nutrition as priorities. Of course there are always blips that will rock your routine: sick kids, holidays, and so on, but provided you get back on track as soon as possible, then it is just that—a blip, not a blockage.

√ Give yourself a decent and well-earned pat on the back for getting here in one piece. Pregnancy is a challenging journey, especially for those over 35.

√ Celebrate your incredible body that has served you so well during pregnancy, birth and beyond.

√ Be patient with yourself.

√ Stay healthy, keep smiling and encourage all those other mums and 'mums-in-waiting' you know to get active.
I wish you well.
Suzy

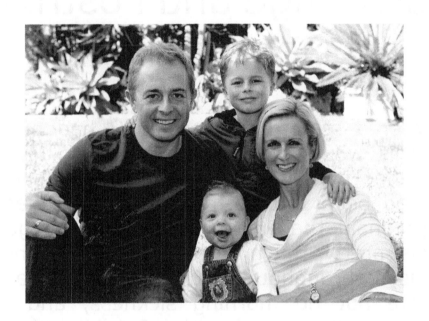

Chapter 9

My Journey Through IVF, Miscarriage and Postnatal Depression

When I started this project I had no idea that this would feature in the book. My first pregnancy in 2007 had gone exceedingly well and had been trouble-free. I was fortunate to get pregnant the first time we tried at age 39. It was pretty much a textbook pregnancy. I exercised throughout, had a slight decrease in appetite but no morning sickness, and gave birth naturally to a healthy 3.4 kilos (or 7.5 pounds) boy at 39 weeks. Bingo! I breastfed like a trooper, using a double breast pump to make sure I had enough supply. After reading all the books on the importance of routines for a newborn, I had Ben sleeping through the night at 8 weeks and was back to work (TV newsreading) at 12 weeks. Then my first speed bump appeared.

At about six months I developed postnatal depression. Thinking back on this period in my life, it was as though I gradually just got really down and dark about life. I found it hard to find the positive in anything. I remember sitting on a beach during the summer holidays with my girlfriends and confessing that, despite this gorgeous setting of which I would normally be most appreciative, I was so depressed and sad. It was incongruous with my normal nature, and so I decided to see my family doctor. I hadn't read much about postnatal depression, and, since my first three months as a new mum had gone fairly smoothly, I certainly didn't think a condition like this would sneak up and bite me at six months postpartum. My family doctor picked the signs as soon as I saw her, and said I could choose to treat it with either medication or counselling. I chose counselling and saw a lovely lady for a handful of sessions, some involving my husband. After a few months of getting myself sorted out I seemed to flick back to normal me. So that was my thankfully brief experience of postnatal depression.

I became pregnant for a second time two years later, in May 2009. All the normal factors had aligned to allow me to fall pregnant the instant we started trying: we were on holiday, I was fit and healthy, and we were using an ovulation saliva tester kit to establish the 'right' time. However, even I was pretty blown away by replicating my luck of getting pregnant on the first attempt.

Postnatal depression

Postnatal depression is similar to clinical depression and, according to Plunket New Zealand, affects about 13% of new mums, and can occur at any time in the first year. This is more than just temporarily feeling down or having a bout of 'the blues'. It is when a number of symptoms appear together over a sustained length of time. Symptoms like tiredness, aches and pains, negative thoughts, worry, a low or flat mood, and concentration and thinking difficulties. The most important course of action you can take is to tell someone: don't judge yourself, don't accept this feeling as normal, and most importantly seek help from a professional. Support, counselling and medication can all help recovery.

Helpful websites

www.mothersmatter.co.nz The Postnatal Depression Family/Whanau New Zealand Trust was set up as a charitable trust in 2006 to improve awareness and understanding of postnatal depression and related mental illnesses in pregnancy and after childbirth. The trust hopes women in the community and their families/whanau will feel less isolated and be more able to access help by using this information.

www.plunket.org.nz   PlunketLine
0800-933-922

www.panda.org.au   In an independent, international study, Australia's Post and Antenatal Depression Association (PANDA) was rated as the worldwide website leader for mothers with a postnatal mental illness. The CEO of PANDA, Belinda Horton, says: 'Around one in seven new mothers and one in ten new fathers are diagnosed with postnatal depression and many of them are reluctant to seek help. PANDA's website is often the first, critical contact point that makes it easier for people to get vital information and support in the privacy of their own homes.'

Because of the ease of my first pregnancy two years previously, I felt comfortable telling close family and friends our 'news' within the first six weeks. However, I noticed some marked differences compared with the first time around. This time I was absolutely exhausted in the evenings, to the point of 'hitting the wall' about 6pm and barely being able to eat dinner before crashing into bed. It was as if any energy had been sucked out of me via a large pipe.

I was hungrier than ever and resorted to carrying snack foods in my handbag and having substantial-sized meals. Again, this was different from my first experience of pregnancy, when with Ben I struggled with having any appetite at all—and as I am normally a voracious eater,

I found it most bizarre to be uninterested in food. I felt a bit ripped off, too, as I didn't even have any cravings. Anyway, back to pregnancy number two, which was proceeding quite differently.

My belly started to show a little bulge by my first scan at six weeks, and the scan appeared normal in every respect. The heart beat was strong, the fetus a good length and size. I left the obstetrician's with ticks in all the right boxes and instructions to continue on as normal.

Then at 11 1/2 weeks, two days before my son's second birthday, without warning, it happened. I began to lose my baby. Unbeknown to me, my body had actually been on this course of action probably for two or three weeks and this was its final physical conclusion. But to me it was a sudden and brutal shock. At first I absolutely discounted the possibility that something was wrong. It was just a little bleeding; nothing to worry about. But the next morning there was no doubting something was up. Still believing the baby could be saved, I went for a scan at the obstetrician's. As soon as I saw the ultrasound image on the screen with no visible heartbeat, my heart sank. The doctor then sensitively confirmed my worst fears: 'There is no heartbeat, Suzy, and the baby is not the right size. It probably stopped growing three weeks ago—it should be double that size at this stage. I'm afraid this is not good news.' Still in shock I asked if he could be mistaken. Did he ever get this sort of diagnosis wrong? He offered me the option of a second opinion, but already I knew in my heart that his observations were true.

So there I was, abruptly standing at an abyss, with all my hopes, expectations and love for this baby suddenly wrenched from my grasp. I wanted to stop the world, to rewind the clock: to make this *not* be. The following 24 hours were a blur of mental anguish plus the physical process of my body eliminating the pregnancy that wasn't to be.

I went through the stages of grief. Shock (Is this really happening?), denial (No, no, it's not happening to me!), grief (This is desperately sad), anger (Why me? What have I done to deserve this?), and, finally, understanding and acceptance (It does happen, and it *has* happened. It is common. It is not my fault and I will deal with it.)

In the immediate aftermath I did my own personal farewell to the little baby whom I would never meet, details of which I shall always keep private, but it was a valuable part of my own process of closure.

Miscarriage and the fact that we don't usually know why it has happened will often evoke a desperate search for answers by the woman affected. For me, that meant the start of the 'blame game'. Even though I had been told you are unlikely to find a reason, you start searching for one and examining the minutiae of what you have done over the preceding few weeks. Was it the stress of my 14-year-old dog (and loyal buddy) Jazz dying? Did having a tiny sip of wine on an evening out contribute? Did I eat the right things? Did I do the right exercise, and did I rest enough? The answer to all of the above, based on research and medical opinion, is that it is extremely unlikely that any of those factors played a part in my miscarriage. However, that didn't stop those questions playing on my mind.

Ultimately I found comfort and acceptance in the phrase 'some things are just not meant to be'. Nature is a powerful force, and it had decided that this pregnancy would not proceed for reasons that I will never know. I stood to gain nothing by blaming myself or circumstances that were beyond my control.

What I found myself enveloped in, however, was a huge outpouring of empathy and understanding from family and friends. Women whom I already knew had suffered a miscarriage, or several, shared their intimate stories and recoveries. Women who in the past hadn't revealed to me their loss now opened up and shared their sad experiences. Suddenly I wasn't the only one who had loved and lost, it was friends, family and friends of friends. There's a saying 'a problem shared is a problem halved', and simply being able to express my fears and insecurities around the whole situation with those who understood first-hand what I was going through did much to ease my mind and help my recovery.

Every woman who sadly experiences a miscarriage will react differently. There is no right or wrong way of feeling. It is the strength of the bond you have developed with that baby that will often determine your intensity of grief, not the length of the pregnancy. I did find myself a little wistful when observing other friends' pregnancies that had been around the same date as mine and that thankfully were carrying on as normal. I found myself asking: How will I feel when they have their child? Will I go through the sadness of thinking that could have been me? One of my key life phrases has been 'onwards and upwards', and I was keen to move forward from this loss. Over the next few months I found I became quite pragmatic about it. I focused on getting fit and healthy, and preparing to try again.

Miscarriage

Research shows the chances that your next pregnancy will succeed only drop by 5% after one miscarriage. Although I felt ready to move on after just a few months, it is normal for the grieving process to take around six months, even for women who did not plan their pregnancy. Every woman will travel the journey differently.

If you have experienced a miscarriage and you would like to discuss any aspect of it, don't hesitate to contact a support organisation. Here are some good starter contacts, but if you search online for 'miscarriage + [your location]' you will find a local support group.

Helpful websites

New Zealand

Miscarriage Support Auckland Inc.

Website: www.miscarriage.org.nz

Support Line: NZ +09-378-4060

Email support@miscarriagesupport.org.nz

Australia

National Association of SANDS organisations supporting families who experience miscarriage, stillbirth, neonatal and infant death.

Website: www.sands.org.au

Support Line: Aust +(03)9899-0218

Email: info@sandsvic.org.au Australian

So back to my journey which was about to unfold in a manner that was to prove a challenge at every turn for the next three years.

We waited a few months and started trying again. I was now 41 years old, but I had no real concept of how my fertility might be profoundly affected by my age; after all, in the previous few years I had got pregnant both first times we had tried. We tried for six months with no result, and then decided (with the clock ticking for me and the desire not to have too big a gap between children) that we would go and seek IVF help.

My first appointment was 11 March 2010. We decided to first try a drug that increases the production of eggs, so that each month I'd have more than one attempt of an egg getting fertilised. This was all about increasing my odds. I had all the usual battery of blood tests and scans to check everything was operating as it should be. All came back clear and in working order. My husband also had his sperm tested, again all normal.

So taking this drug involved a protocol of tablets taken orally, then a scan to check egg production, and blood tests followed by trying to conceive in the normal manner, albeit on specific days according to predicted ovulation dates and with more mature eggs coming down the tubes. No joy with the first try, so we tried again for the following two months. By June we decided we would take a big step and give IVF a go. This is a whole lot more involved, with a strict regime of drugs, hormones, injections, egg harvesting, laboratory insemination of the egg to try to make a viable embryo, and, if you're lucky and you get good embryo growth, implantation of those embryos back into a pre-prepared receptive uterus. With a wing and a prayer that Nature will take over and do its thing from then on.

Dealing with IVF quickly becomes your life. You have emotionally and financially invested in the outcome. You hear all sorts of well-meaning comments from friends like 'it will happen if you just relax/it will happen if you just take a holiday/stop working/try acupuncture/try a special diet from my naturopath' and so on. They are all well meaning, for sure, but a vulnerable person, who is just wanting to tip the scales and get some biological luck, can't help thinking: 'What if I did those things? Would it help?' Quite frankly, you are prepared to give almost anything a go to try to get yourself out of this predicament.

At this point in my journey I was still reasonably optimistic that I would overcome this temporary lack of luck and that I would get pregnant again. I was throwing everything I could at it: emotional energy, money to employ the best science, and looking after myself with careful diet and exercise. I had cut out coffee, didn't touch alcohol when 'in cycle', and I had signed up for regular acupuncture sessions. My first harvest (a medical procedure where a doctor extracts the eggs from your ovaries) went well, with 18 inseminated and 13 progressing in the laboratory to fertilisation stage. Then it is a case of waiting to see the embryos' progress into day five blastocysts, before you make a decision on whether you will do a fresh embryo transfer with some and freeze others for a transfer at a later date (Fig.9.1). Every blastocyst represented a chance of a baby in my mind, and I had eight from this first cycle. Surely I must get some success from this?

Then followed a month-by-month process of preparing my body to have a series of embryo transfers (which means making sure your hormones are at the most conducive levels for pregnancy), blood tests (sometimes daily), and a waiting game each month to find out if the blastocysts (there are often two put back at once) have taken. So it is a continuous cycle of hope, expectation, optimism, disappointment and despair, which affects you to varying levels depending on how many blastocysts you have left, whether they are rated as good quality, and your powers of endurance.

I have always thought of myself as having a reasonably strong character, able to cope with the trials and tribulations that life inevitably throws at each and every one of us, but dealing with infertility has tested me in ways I never would have ever imagined. It makes you ask some very fundamental questions about why you want children; your expectations of having a family of a certain size and why you can't just be happy with one child. I found writing a journal the only way I could deal with this baffling array of soul-probing questions. That's not to say that the journal actually made sense—it was often just pages expressing an outpouring of grief, a diatribe of 'Why me? Why not...?', and pleading for some fairness. Writing down my fears helped me expose them, and that seemed to make them a little easier to deal with and at least keep them in perspective. It allowed me to carry on working and to keep the infertility journey just between myself, my husband and close family. As each attempt at success came and went and the 'temporary bad luck' started to ebb into years, it became apparent that this quite clearly wasn't temporary. It was what is termed 'secondary infertility', and it hurt a lot. I could never have anticipated how much our desire to add just one more child to our family would cause such a roller-coaster of emotional turmoil, and I am also not one to give up easily.

I exhausted the supply of embryos with the first cycle and then embarked on a whole new cycle of IVF. This involved more drugs, more diarising, more putting our lives on hold to try to chance our luck at biological success. I was also seeing a specialist IVF counsellor by now; a lovely lady who was aptly named Joi. She saw my tears and bitter despair when a transfer had failed, we discussed the intimate details of how progressing on this journey may never actually get me the result I wanted. That was hard to hear. But talking to this counsellor and dumping down my thoughts in a journal, combined with a totally supportive husband, were the essential tools I needed to traverse this grim reality.

During the cycles and transfers, I was also investigating everything I could to increase my chances. I was put on an increased drug regime called the Colorado protocol, which had produced some success for some patients. I also had my uterus and fallopian tubes re-checked and flushed with a solution that again was meant to increase fertility chances. I had come this far, why not do everything possible?

It was January 2011 now, and I had just turned 43. I remember having a conversation about my chances with fertility treatment and it went something like this: 'At your age the chance of conceiving using IVF is about 5–10%.' Well remembering those statistics now it seems pretty grim, but here is the strange thing: I didn't hear that the actual failure rate is about 90–95%; I just heard the positive percentage. That's what hope and optimism do to you. When you want something badly you'll find a way to interpret the facts that suits your ideal outcome. I subsequently learnt the real meaning of that conversation of percentages.

My second IVF cycle got 12 eggs with 9 fertilised, 3 replaced fresh on day three, and only 1 blastocyst frozen. Again a negative result from both the fresh replacements and the frozen one a month on. The feeling you have when you discover that your body isn't pregnant after all this effort is hard to explain. It's a mixture of shock, anger at yourself, a feeling your body has let you down, anger at the science having failed you, and the injustice of it all, which with time slowly fades to frustration, intense disappointment and then eventually the question 'What next?'

My third IVF cycle also produced 12 eggs, 9 fertilised, 2 implanted and only 1 frozen for future use.

By March 2011 I was like a pin cushion and was very adept at giving myself injections. I had the drugs regimen totally sorted, and, despite there being a cocktail of pills to take from day to day, my body seemed to cope pretty well with minimal side-effects. Each time I did a replacement we got a computer image printout of the actual embryos they replaced. I still have some of those. You cherish them, putting your hopes and dreams into the image that this will be *the one.*

The wait between having an embryo replaced and the 10 days until the blood test to show any sign of pregnancy is excruciating. Your mind plays tricks on you. You treat yourself with velvet gloves, not doing anything too physical. Being as gentle on your body as possible, giving yourself the best possible chance, and all the while it's a calendar countdown until you are booked for that crucial blood test. I got very friendly with the ladies at my local laboratory. This is good and bad.

Good if you are in a hopeful and optimistic mood, bad if you are worried and feeling sensitive about what might be the outcome from that little vial of blood they take. And then there is the phone call.

Mine were always timed for about 12pm, when the blood results from the laboratory got back to the clinic. I'd usually be at work, but nervously waiting for the phone to ring and the result to be revealed. I often held my breath. I usually found a little quiet room, which was just as well, as the number of times I had negative results I do not want to even think about. My stomach would sink and I'd be numb. I would ring Tim and give him the news, and then I would have to gather myself up, take a deep breath and go out and greet the world again as though nothing had happened. It was tough, there's no denying it. I wouldn't wish it on anyone. Then my period would arrive and I would be visibly reminded of the reality of failure.

About this time my husband and I had some pretty in-depth talks about whether we were done with trying. There is no doubt we wanted another child, but we did consider the reality that maybe it was just not ever meant to be. Maybe regardless of the best intentions and the best treatment money could buy, we were just not going to be successful.

I was being forced to accept that, unlike other areas of my life in which I had a

484

reasonable amount of control over my destiny, in this one area I had none. Nothing I did seemed to be helping. Time was passing. My natural optimism had been replaced with a grinding pessimism, with optimism just in occasional bursts. Was this process that had already spanned two and half years changing me as a person? Undoubtedly, yes is the answer. It is very difficult to understand infertility unless you have been faced with it yourself. There is a starkness, a loneliness and a sense of futility that is hard to share, and probably even harder to grasp for those from the outside. I guess that's why women who have faced this find solace in discussing their situation with others in the same boat, although it has to be in a general sense, as with infertility treatments the journey is so specific to the individual.

Secondary infertility can really challenge on your relationship, too. It affects you both, but in different ways. It can pull you together, but also split you apart. It's an undercurrent, a day-to-day strain, not something short-term that blows over. I still don't know how Tim and I got through these three years really. I guess we dug deep and empathised with the way each of us was reacting from day to day.

Despite feeling pretty battle-worn, we embarked on a fourth attempt. This time we tried a different regimen. After implantation I was taking intramuscular injections every night and a much more elaborate drug regimen. The injections were painful. I couldn't do them myself, so Tim had to be trained to give them. Sometimes they'd be relatively easy, other times I'd yelp with pain. The hormone in oil that I was injecting often formed a hard lump in the buttock muscle, which was sore to touch, and made large areas on my buttocks and down my legs go numb. Again, I wouldn't wish this on anyone. It is surprising what you will endure if you think it will help you achieve a positive result, and this far into the journey I wasn't about to let physical pain get in the way.

I waited anxiously for the call from the clinic after having my first pregnancy blood test 10 days after embryo transfer. It doesn't sound long to wait—just 10 days—but it felt like a lifetime. Tim and I met at a local shopping centre car park and we sat in the car together to get the news via phone. I can still remember the sheer elation from hearing 'congratulations'. I burst into tears, scarcely believing what I had heard. We just felt blessed and oh so lucky.

The next few weeks were a whirlwind of absorbing the news and keeping as quiet as possible about it. We knew there were hurdles to get past, and we just wanted to make it through those first 12 weeks. I had blood tests every week to check that the level of pregnancy hormone was progressing. It was on the chart, it was smack bang centre, and it was increasing. I was thrilled and felt as though all the hard work and waiting were finally over. I felt we had got our reward for being so patient and persistent for the past two and a half years. My mind started planning ahead. When would the baby be due? When would I stop work? When should I tell my friends? I got out my pram and scrubbed it down. I started thinking which bedroom I would convert for the baby's room. We were in planning mode, and we were so grateful to be on the positive side of the tracks again. My next few blood tests showed a normal increase in pregnancy hormone, and given my first pregnancy had progressed normally I was optimistic that this, too, would be successful.

On 7 February 2012, I received a call from the clinic. The last blood test had not shown the kind of rise that would normally be expected. However there was nothing to panic about, but perhaps, they suggested, I would like to come in for a scan to allay any concerns. I was there within a few hours. It was a cruel discovery. The baby had not grown sufficiently for the date of gestation; there was no heartbeat to be seen. It was grim news. I was devastated, and so was Tim. To get this close after all our trying and then to have it ripped away was unbelievably sad. Words can't really express the depths I sank to. I decided to have D&C (dilation and curettage) procedure. It all unfolded like a bad dream, really. Booked in, process done, end of story. Back to ground zero. We had testing done on the embryo, and several weeks later we were told that the pregnancy had ended because of a chromosomal abnormality. The sort that meant the pregnancy was never likely to continue and it had probably stopped growing at about six weeks.

This time I *really* needed counselling. You console yourself with thoughts like 'Oh well, it wasn't meant to be, it's a common reason for miscarriage' and anything else you can dream up to soften the blow. One of the articles I read simply said, 'recognising that goodness is not always rewarded, and that bad things happen to good people is sobering and may be difficult to accept'. About now is when many people would stop and say enough is enough. I did consider it, but I had five frozen embryos left. I had to continue. How could I leave embryos in a test tube without ever knowing the outcome?

And so the journey continued. Another replacement cycle with two replaced; two that were of high grade and I felt terribly positive about; but the result was negative.

Finally it came down to the last three embryos. In my mind I was now getting very close to the end of the journey once and for all. With the last three all transferred at once, I was not optimistic at all; in fact, I was fatalistic if anything. I was tired of trying, tired of getting hopeful only to have everything shattered in a one-word result. Tim and I met at a quiet café to get the results on the phone. I don't think I could speak when the lady from the clinic actually said 'congratulations'. The tears came fast and didn't stop for quite a while. But this time, instead of pure elation, there was incredible anxiety and worry that it would go the same way as the previous result. I couldn't bear to think of dealing with that again. I received each blood test with the same nervousness. The experience couldn't have been more of a contrast to my first pregnancy, when I believed everything would go right, and thankfully it did. Back then, five years before, I was bulletproof. This time I was 44, at the end of a long emotional road, and a bag of nerves that at any moment my slim grip on a second baby would be taken from me.

I had weekly scans for the first 10 weeks (which is far more frequently than usual) to keep my anxiety at bay. Every scan was another slight relief, but my real milestones were the 12-week stage and then the 20-week stage. I had nausea and tiredness, probably not helped by my being a bag of nerves at every twinge and turn. I was told not to exercise aside from walking, and having endured a fairly rough ride to get to this point I didn't tempt fate by doing anything different. I bought a heart-rate monitor and made sure my daily walks of about 45 minutes were not taking me to an overheated or sweaty level. If I had used velvet gloves previously to look after myself, this time they were padded times a thousand. I remember my specialist saying very sagely that given what I had been through the anxiety over this pregnancy was not going to end until I had a live baby in my arms, and he was right. It was tough not doing much exercise in the first 12 weeks, but it was for a very good reason. At three months all the scans and baby growth were positive, so I could proceed as per a normal pregnancy. Having a balanced programme of strengthening, modified cardiovascular exercise and stretching made me feel normal again.

In summary, the journey my husband and I have been on is not one I would wish on anyone. However, we have been so lucky that in the end we got a positive result. It has definitely changed me; I hope for the better, in that I now have a very comprehensive understanding of infertility and the trials and tribulations a couple can go through trying to have a baby. Some people aren't so lucky, and I could easily have been one of those, too. Towards the end of my IVF attempts I was facing that very reality and I know it would have been difficult to accept, but in saying that I guess that I would have coped, eventually. You never say goodbye to infertility—it's still something, once experienced, that lives with you. I know that despite the effort, the attention to detail, the velvet gloves and the hopes and prayers, ultimately in my mind it comes down to biology. It is either going to work or it won't, and provided all your other bits are functioning it is the viability of the egg and sperm that ultimately determines success. We know we are extraordinarily lucky, and this last pregnancy was a wee miracle.

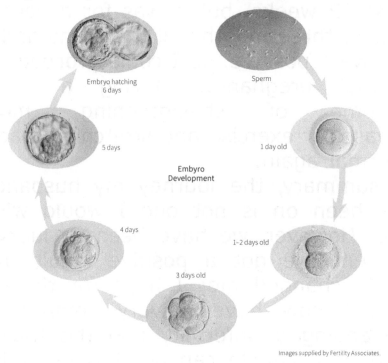

Images supplied by Fertility Associates.

Fig.9.1

Appendix A

The Bare Essentials Routine

There are bound to be times during your nine months of pregnancy when tiredness or other minor symptoms mean that you can't physically bring yourself to do an exercise workout of even moderate intensity. That's okay. Most importantly it is crucial that you *listen* to your body at these times and *don't push yourself.* There is likely to be a very good reason for it: not the least of which is that your body is spending a lot of effort and energy developing another human being. The first and third trimesters are often the time when you will get waves of tiredness: the former often due to the increase in pregnancy hormones, changes in circulation, and other physiological adaptations to being newly pregnant; and the latter due to disturbed sleep and the daily effort of carrying those necessary extra baby kilos.

So what are your alternatives? You could do nothing or you could do this Bare Essentials routine. I am not going to call it a workout, as it will not get you even close to breaking a sweat. It is more a series of moves and stretches designed specifically for pregnancy that will take you about 15 minutes to complete in total, and provide you with a sense of achievement and a feeling of wellbeing without the exertion.

You will need a Swiss ball and a space of about 2 metres square.

1 Foot pedals on the spot

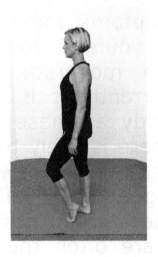

With your feet hip-distance apart, press through the toes to do alternate heel lifts. Continue for 1 minute. This exercise is good for circulation.

2 Pelvic tilts

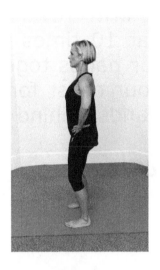

From a neutral stance, tuck your buttocks under, pull your belly button towards your spine, and lift up your pelvic floor muscles. Repeat 10 times.

3 Shoulder rolls and chest-opener

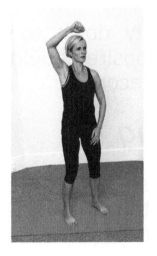 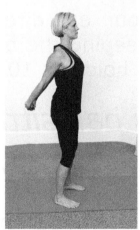

Lift both shoulders up, then roll them back and down, continue circling and increasing the movement to full-arm reverse circles with a bent elbow. Repeat 10 times each side.

Then clasp your hands together behind your back and press your chest forwards as you try to elevate your hands behind you.

4 Neck stretch

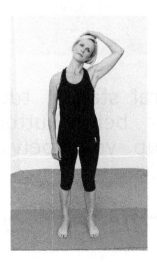

Drop your ear directly down towards your shoulder, keeping the opposite shoulder pressed down, and hold for 10 seconds.

5 Swiss ball sitting

If you feel unsteady sitting on the ball, take your feet slightly wider than hip distance apart to provide a more stable base.

a Hip rotations

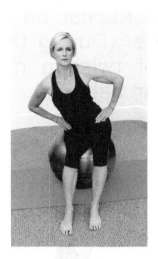

Sitting on the apex of a Swiss ball, with your feet flat on the floor, roll your hips in a full circle. Do this 10 times in one direction, then repeat in reverse.

b Upper body twist

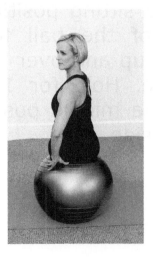

From a stable sitting position with an upright upper body, bring one hand across to the outside of the opposite thigh and turn around and look behind you—perform the rotation movement slowly. Repeat on the other side, 2 times on each side. (During the third trimester, limit the range of twisting motion so you do not compress your baby.)

c Side flexion

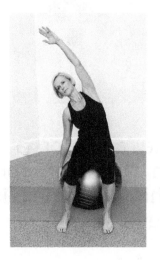

From a stable sitting position, put one arm down the side of the ball for stability, and extend the other up and over your head as you bend to the side. Hold for 10 seconds, then return back to the middle position, and repeat on the opposite side.

d Hamstring stretch

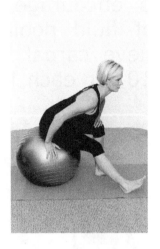

Extend one leg out, foot flexed and knee straight, then bend forward from the hips with a flat back and without twisting. Check that your shoulders are parallel to the floor, and put your hands and weight onto the bent knee. Just go as far as necessary in order to feel a stretch on the underside of the extended leg. Repeat on the other side.

e Ankle and wrist rotations

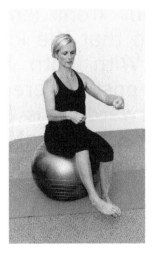

These are particularly relevant during the third trimester to encourage good circulation and prevention of fluid pooling in the lower limbs, also to relieve carpal tunnel discomfort in the wrist. Do 10 for each limb.

Transition

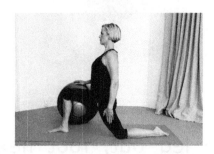

From sitting, lower yourself slowly until you are kneeling on the floor; use the ball or a chair alongside for stability. You may wish to put a folded towel on the floor to cushion your knee.

6 Hip flexor stretch

Make sure your front leg is extended far enough forward so that the knee is at 90° and not over-flexed. With both hips parallel and your upper-body posture erect, press the hip of the rear leg forward. It is a small move and the upper body stays upright. Repeat on other side.

7 Deep squat

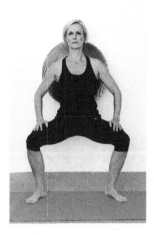

With stable back support from a solid couch, a wall or a Swiss ball against the wall, assume a deep squat position. You are best to get into this position from kneeling. Lean your body weight back into the support—your leg muscles should not be working hard in this position. Hold for 30–60 seconds. If you have knee joint problems, then skip this position.

8 Seated butterfly stretch

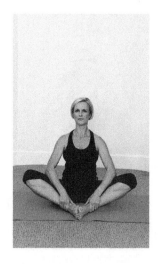

Sit on the floor, again with back support, bring the soles of your feet together, and let your bent knees flop out. Hold for 30–60 seconds.

9 Prayer stretch

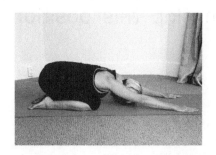

From your hands and knees, extend your hands well out on the floor in front of you, then pull back and lower your body until you feel a stretch through your arms and chest.

Keep your head in line with your spine or rest your forehead on the ground. Hold for 20–30 seconds.

10 Half-lying or sitting relaxation

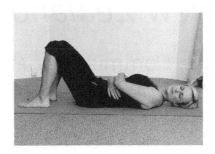

You may wish to finish by practising some deep breathing as a form of relaxation. Sit or lie in a comfortable, supported position, with your shoulders down and relaxed. Concentrate on breathing slowly and deeply, letting the air fill your lungs from the bottom, with your lower ribs and stomach swelling out as you inhale, then gently dropping back as you exhale. As you complete a set of 10, try to get each one a little deeper and taking a little longer than the previous one, but don't force it. You may find wrapping your arms loosely around your lower ribs helps you focus on getting your breaths deeper, lower and slower.

Well done!

References

Documents

Australia/New Zealand

Australian Sports Commission, *Pregnancy in Sport: Guidelines for the Australian Sporting Industry,* ASC, 2002.

Families Commission, *The Kiwi Nest: 60 Years of Change in New Zealand Families,* Families Commission, 2008.

Kruger JA, Murphy BA and Thompson S, 'Childbirth and Sportswomen: The Perception of Obstetric Caregivers', *Vision – A Journal of Nursing,* Vol 14 (2), February 2007.

Kruger JA, Dietz HP and Murphy BA, 'Pelvic Floor Function in Elite Nulliparous Athletes', *Ultrasound in Obstetrics and Gynecology,* 30:81–85, 2007.

Les Mills International, *Pregnancy Guides Group Fitness Classes for PUMP™, BODYBALANCE™ and BODYVIVE™,* Les Mills International, 2012.

Ministry of Health NZ, *Eating for Healthy Breastfeeding Women/NgāKai Totika mā te Ūkaipō*, 2013.

Ministry of Health, *Food and Nutrition Guidelines for Pregnant and Breastfeeding Women: A Background Paper,* Ministry of Health, Wellington, 2006.

Ministry of Health (New Zealand) and Australian Government (joint document), *Nutrient Reference Values for Australia and New Zealand, including Recommended Dietary Intakes,* endorsed by the NHMRC on 9 September 2005, published 2006.

Miscarriage Support Auckland Inc, *Understanding Miscarriage* (brochure), October 2008.

New South Wales Department of Sport and Recreation, *Active Community Guide: Mum's the Word Exercise During Pregnancy,* August 2001.

Sapsford RR, Richardson CA, Cooper DH, Markwell SJ and Jull GA, 'Co-activation of the Abdominal and Pelvic Floor Muscles During

Voluntary Exercises', *Neurology and Urodynamics,* 20:31–42, 2001.

Sports Medicine Australia, *Statement on the Benefits and Risks of Exercise During Pregnancy,* March 2002, endorsed by the Women's Health Committee of the Royal Australian and New Zealand College of Obstetricians and Gynaecologists (RANZCOG), November 2004.

Statistics New Zealand, *Births and Deaths: Median Age of Women Giving Birth in New Zealand,* March 2009.

Statistics New Zealand, *Births and Deaths: Year Ended June 2011 Median Age of First Birth NZ Women,* June 2011.

Victorian Government, 'Better Health Channel Factsheet: Pregnancy and Exercise', May 2008.

Victorian Government, 'Better Health Channel Factsheet: Pregnancy and Sport', May 2009.

Wainwright, Torfrida (for the New Zealand Continence Association), *Reviewing the Need*

for Current Organisation of Continence Services,
2006.

United Kingdom

Royal College of Obstetricians and
Gynaecologists, *Patient Information:
Recreational Exercise and Pregnancy,* RCOG,
September 2006.

Royal College of Obstetricians and
Gynaecologists, *Statement on Exercise in
Pregnancy,* RCOG, January 2006.

United States

American College of Obstetricians and
Gynaecologists, *Guidelines for Exercise During
Pregnancy and Postpartum,* ACOG, 2002.

American College of Obstetricians and
Gynaecologists (ACOG), *Patient Education:
Exercise During Pregnancy,* June 2003.

506

Canada

Society of Obstetricians and Gynaecologists of Canada and Canadian Society for Exercise Physiology (joint authors), *Exercise in Pregnancy and the Postpartum Period,* SOGC/CSEP Joint Clinical Practice Guideline, No 129, June 2003.

France

The Organisation for Economic Cooperation and Development (OECD), *Doing Better For Families Report,* OECD Publishing, 2011.

The Organisation for Economic Cooperation and Development (OECD), *Family Database,* OECD Publishing, 2012.

Books

Adamany, Karrie, *Post Pregnancy Pilates: An Essential Guide for a Fit Body After Baby,* Penguin, New York, 2005.

Aiken, Suzy and Holdom, Karen, *Healthy Body, Healthy Mind,* HarperCollins, Auckland, 1997.

Baker, Cherry, *Pregnancy and Fitness,* A & C Black, London, 2006.

Bell, Anita Weil, *Get Your Body Back,* St Martins, New York, 2002.

Bryne, Helen, *Exercise After Pregnancy,* Celestial Arts, Berkeley, 2001.

Clapp James F III, MD, *Exercising Through Your Pregnancy,* Addicus Books, Omaha, Nebraska, 2002.

Corey, Kathy, *Total Core Fitness: Stronger, Leaner and Fitter to the Core,* Barron's Educational Series, New York, 2006.

Craig, Colleen, *Strength Training On The Ball: A Pilates Approach to Optimal Strength and Balance,* Healing Arts Press, Rochester, Vermont, 2005.

Frediani, Paul, *Powersculpt: The Women's Body Sculpting and Weight Training Workout Using*

508

the Exercise Ball, Healthy Living Books, New York, 2003.

Hargraves, Fiona Thomas, *Fit and Fabulous—For Life After Babies,* Allen & Unwin, Crows Nest, NSW, 2009.

Haas, Elson M, MD, *Staying Healthy with Nutrition—The Complete Guide to Diet and Nutritional Medicine,* Celestial Arts, Berkeley, 1992.

Pullon, Sue and Benn, Cheryl, *The New Zealand Pregnancy Book: A Guide to Pregnancy, Birth and a Baby's First Three Months,* 3rd ed., Bridget Williams Books, Wellington, 2008.

Wiess, RE, *The Everything Pregnancy Fitness Book,* F+W Publications, Avon, Montana, 2004.

Useful Websites

www.nzfsa.govt.nz
www.foodstandards.gov.au
www.foodsmart.govt.nz
www.foodauthority.nsw.gov.au
www.healthed.govt.nz

www.health.gov.au

www.thewomens.org.au/healthyeatingforpregna
 ncy

www.pregnancyexercise.co.nz

www.betterhealth.vic.gov.au

www.babycentre.com.au

www.babycentre.co.nz

www.babycentre.co.uk

www.fertilityassociates.co.nz

www.sands.org.au

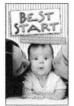
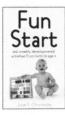
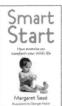
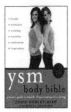

Suzy Clarkson qualified as a physiotherapist in 1988. She then went on to an extensive and successful career in broadcasting, completing a postgraduate diploma in broadcast journalism (England 2002) before returning to New Zealand to host Prime News for six years. In the 1990s she qualified as an ACE (American Council of Exercise) personal trainer and taught a variety of group fitness classes. Her first book on general health and wellbeing, *Healthy Body Healthy Mind,* was published in 1997. She has also created and produced four aerobic videos: *Fit Kit, Fit Kit 2, Fitness Plus* and *Move It.* Suzy is a minor investor in Les Mills International. She currently lives in Auckland with her two sons Ben and Toby, husband Tim and dog Roxy and works as a Corporate Affairs Manager.

Back Cover Material

'Excellent ... likely to become the defining book of exercise in pregnancy.'
Dr Derek Souter FRCOG, obstetrician

Many older women spend months, if not years, trying for motherhood, then endure an anxious pregnancy wondering if they are eating and exercising properly. Fitness expert Suzy Clarkson has been there. Her first pregnancy at the age of 39 was relatively trouble-free, but trying to get pregnant again a few years later was very different. Following extensive fertility treatment, she gave birth to her second child at the age of 45.

Qualified in physiotherapy, Suzy has now devised a practical guide to assist women through their pregnancies, supported by her own experiences of motherhood in the frank diary entries scattered throughout the book. The easy-to-follow fitness programme will take you through each trimester, showing suitable exercises and suggesting how to develop healthy habits and good nutrition to achieve a safe outcome, a successful childbirth and a speedy recovery afterwards. The book is fully illustrated with step-by-step photographs showing the exercises in detail. The information she provides is based on the latest research, and is endorsed by leading specialists in obstetrics and fertility.

But the book is more than its exercises. Suzy is a 'real mum' who offers encouragement and a compassionate helping hand to all mothers. *Fit for Birth and Beyond* is the guide you can trust and use with confidence.